AF572591

SYNCOPE

Volume 18 in the Series

Major Problems in Neurology
SIR JOHN WALTON, TD, MD, DSc, FRCP
Consulting Editor

OTHER MONOGRAPHS IN THE SERIES

Barnett, Foster and Hudgson: **Syringomyelia**
Dubowitz and Brooke: **Muscle Biopsy: A Modern Approach**
Pallis and Lewis: **The Neurology of Gastrointestinal Disease**
Hutchinson and Acheson: **Strokes**
Gubbay: **The Clumsy Child**
Hankinson and Banna: **Pituitary and Parapituitary Tumours**
Donaldson: **Neurology of Pregnancy**
Behan and Currie: **Clinical Neuroimmunology**
Harper: **Myotonic Dystrophy**
Cartlidge and Shaw: **Head Injury**
Lisak and Barchi: **Myasthenia Gravis**
Porter: **Epilepsy: 100 Elementary Principles**
Johnson, Lambie and Spalding: **Neurocardiology: The Interrelationships between Dysfunction in the Nervous and Cardiovascular Systems**
Parkes: **Sleep and its Disorders**
Hopkins: **Headache: Problems in Diagnosis and Management**
Wood and Anderson: **Neurological Infections**
Critchley: **Neurological Emergencies**

SYNCOPE

R. T. ROSS, M.D., F.R.C.P.

Department of Medicine (Neurology)
The University of Manitoba, Health Sciences Centre,
Winnipeg, Manitoba, CANADA

1988
W. B. Saunders Company
London · Philadelphia · Toronto · Sydney · Tokyo

W. B. Saunders Company 24–28 Oval Road
London NW1 7DX, England

West Washington Square
Philadelphia, PA 19105, USA

1 Goldthorne Avenue
Toronto, Ontario M8Z 5T9, Canada

ABP Australia Ltd
44–50 Waterloo Road
North Ryde, NSW 2113
Australia

Harcourt Brace Jovanovich Japan Inc.
Ichibancho Central Building, 22–1 Ichibancho
Chiyoda-ku, Tokyo 102, Japan

First published 1988

Filmset by Eta Services (Typesetters) Ltd, Beccles, Suffolk
Printed and bound in Great Britain by Mackays of Chatham Ltd.

British Library Cataloguing in Publication Data

Ross, R. T.
Syncope.
1. Man. Fainting
I. Title II. Series
616.8

ISBN 0-7020-1326-9

Contents

Foreword

It may at first sight seem surprising to find a monograph on the topic of syncope being published in a series of works on *Major Problems in Neurology*. However, a number of earlier volumes in this series have concentrated upon that borderline which so clearly exists between neurological medicine and surgery, on the one hand, and other branches of internal medicine and surgery on the other. Thus the series has included books on the neurological manifestations of gastrointestinal disease and on neurocardiology, to quote but two examples. Syncope is a phenomenon which so often enters into the differential diagnosis of epilepsy in patients presenting at neurological clinics that I believe the publication of a monograph on this topic to be timely, and I have no doubt that this clear and comprehensive account, succinctly written by Dr Robert Ross, will be helpful to many neurologists but also to cardiologists, physicians in internal medicine and paediatricians, among others. Dr Ross is, of course, a senior and distinguished Canadian neurologist who has for many years edited the *Canadian Journal of the Neurological Sciences*. He has deployed his literary and editorial skills in writing this monograph in a compact and economical style which has not in my view impaired in any way its readability. As a practising neurologist myself, I have learned a great deal from it, and the care that Dr Ross has exercised in surveying and summarizing important facts from the relevant literature has resulted in my learning of a number of rare but nevertheless important syndromes giving rise to fainting with which I was not previously familiar. I feel sure that many readers of this interesting work will share my view. The clinical descriptions given throughout the book are enlivened by an enlightened discussion of the underlying pathophysiology of the attacks and cogent advice on drug treatment and other aspects of management is offered. I welcome this book as a most worthy addition to the series.

John Walton
Oxford

Preface

Only 3% of the adult population will faint. If appropriate investigation is negative, the faint is not a harbinger of brain or heart disease. The wonder is not why this proportion of the population faints, but why doesn't everyone.

Man standing erect and standing still is on the brink of vasomotor collapse. The venous pressure measured from the dorsum of the foot while standing is sufficient to lift blood to the right atrium without the pumping action of the leg muscles. However, the gradient is just sufficient and varies up to 10 mmH_2O from person-to-person when the measurements are made from the same site. This may help to explain the individual propensity to faint. Diminished right-heart filling pressure is a probable major contributor to the cause of death in crucifixion.

The other side of the circulation in its normal responses can contribute to fainting. Fear or startle produces peripheral vasoconstriction, and increased pulse rate, pressure and blood pressure. The former reduces peripheral venous pressure and thereby right-heart filling. The baroreceptor-mediated responses to these changes in pulse and blood pressure include at times excessive muscle arteriolar and artery vasodilatation, venous dilatation and diminished venous return, and a bradycardia that seems fixed and unresponsive to the ensuing hypotension.

With these sensitive and reciprocal arterial and venous contributions to the stability of the circulation it is not surprising that a host of diseases in many different organs may be characterized by fainting.

Much less stressful situations than prolonged standing or sudden fright can also provoke a faint.

The thin adolescent who faints or nearly faints everytime he stands up quickly and the weightlifter who faints after lifting 250 kg have both stressed physiological systems that need not be diseased but merely overcome at the moment.

The writing of this book has been greatly assisted by Sir John Walton, the series editor. His ideas and criticisms are excellent, he has always been open to new approaches, and I am very grateful.

Katharine Hinton, senior editor, Baillière Tindall Limited, Harcourt Brace Jovanovich is the person every author wants as editor. She is helpful, prompt, to the point and makes the whole process much smoother.

Without Gail Landry, as always, this work would have been impossible. She has retrieved in excess of 1000 references from the Library of the University of Manitoba, Faculty of Medicine, kept them accessible, typed and corrected the manuscript more than once.

Angela Ross, as proof reader of English composition, grammar, and spelling has been indispensible and I am most appreciative.

R. T. Ross

1

The Problem, Patient Evaluation and Diagnostic Methods

Syncope (from the Greek, meaning *to strike, beat, cut off, weary*) is a reversible, temporary, loss of consciousness due to a qualitative or quantitative disturbance of cerebral blood flow. Fainting is a synonymous word with historically more benign connotations.

Syncope, at the least, is a nuisance, inconvenient, uncomfortable, and embarrassing. At the worst, it is dangerous, may be bone breaking and be the premonition of death (Friedberg, 1973). Absent cerebral perfusion for 2–3 seconds causes pre-syncopal sensations and after 10 seconds unconsciousness results (Harvey *et al.*, 1982). With a fall in mean systemic blood pressure below 70 mmHg and the consequent fall in cerebral blood flow to, or below, 30 ml per 100 g of tissue per minute, syncope is about to occur.

A host of varied disorders may present with fainting as a first symptom. These include: diseases of cardiac muscle, valve, conduction, rhythm and outflow obstruction; pulmonary vascular disease and increased intrathoracic pressure; faulty venous return, increased peripheral vascular capacity and abnormal peripheral vascular responses to physiological stimuli; inappropriate nervous stimuli or inhibition of the heart and adverse responses to the normal functions of swallowing or voiding. In addition, such qualitative abnormalities as hypoglycaemia, hypoxia, and hypocapnia are important.

Each of these abnormalities may have its own characteristic history. Some of these are: the child who faints on effort as do others in his family, the teenager who faints when he stands up quickly, the young female adult who faints on effort, and those who faint on a change of position whether upright or lying down.

Some patients who faint have an abnormal response to minor medical interference and instrumentation. These include fainting from ear, eye, thoat and mouth examinations, from venesection ('at the sight of blood'), and from proctoscopic, rectal, prostatic, and vaginal examinations.

Coughing, sneezing, swallowing (hot, cold or body temperature solids or liquids), micturition, vomiting, defaecation, during sexual intercourse or sleeping (producing asystole long enough that one would have fainted if awake), as well as trigeminal or glossopharyngeal neuralgia, and angina pectoris may all provoke a faint. Basilar migraine, posterior fossa arteriosclerosis, and atlanto-occipital junction diseases may have fainting as a common symptom.

Fainting after prolonged bed rest, a debilitating illness or loss of weight in contrast to the faint in physically well (or over-trained) athletes and weightlifters must have very different mechanisms. As the autonomic nervous system decays *de novo* or as part of a diffuse nervous disease, the characteristic faint is associated with rapid standing, after meals, and hot days.

The largest and most benign group of fainters is probably that associated with blood donations, the sight, sound, or smell of something unpleasant, prolonged standing at attention and children who faint in response to sudden, unexpected pain (occasionally with the same history in other family members).

The 'vapours' or faint popular with Victorian ladies of a certain social class seems to have disappeared. Perhaps less restrictive corsetting, higher haemoglobin, and a more direct approach to unpleasant situations has abolished this phenomenon.

The success rate in establishing an aetiological diagnosis in syncope is poor. Even in the hands of a group of physicians as experienced and knowledgeable as Kapoor *et al.* (1983), a diagnosis was made in only half of 204 patients. In comparison to epilepsy, the customary and obvious investigative steps are less distinct and often less revealing. There is a high probability that an adult with a first epileptic seizure will be diagnosed, offered specific treatment, and obtain control of his symptom or treatment of his disease. Another patient with a single syncope stands a good chance of receiving neither diagnosis nor treatment and no advice on what to do or avoid in the future.

SCOPE OF THE PROBLEM

The Framingham Study included a 26-year survey of 5209 subjects, evaluated bi-annually, and revealed some information on fainting. The morbidity and mortality associated with an isolated syncope was determined. Syncope was defined as a 'transient loss of consciousness in the absence of prior or concurrent neurological, coronary, or other cardiovascular disease stigmata'. They found no statistically significant difference in the incidence of stroke or myocardial infarction in those who had an isolated syncopal attack compared to those who did not. Further, syncope in the absence of prior or recurrent neurological, coronary, or other overt cardiovascular disease manifestations was not associated with increased morbidity or mortality. The study suggested that isolated syncope was not a frequent indicator of covert cerebrovascular disease or risk of stroke. More than 75% of the subjects had a single attack only. In the entire 26 years of surveillance at least one syncopal episode was reported by 71 (3%) of the men and 101 (3.5%) of the women (Savage *et al.*, 1985).

Syncope is predominantly a disease of the aged and as the population matures one can expect to see more syncopal patients (Brody, 1984, 1985). C. Miller Fisher (Fisher, 1979) reported his lifetime experience with syncope up to 1979. This included 111 patients with an average age of 62, the oldest was 90. One of the common products of fainting at this age is hip fracture. Figure 1.1 shows the projected incidence of hip fracture by age. While osteoporosis, failing vision, agility and balance, are important causes, fainting also contributes.

HOW GOOD ARE THE DIAGNOSTIC METHODS?

Wayne (1961) reported a retrospective study of 510 patients and found only five with

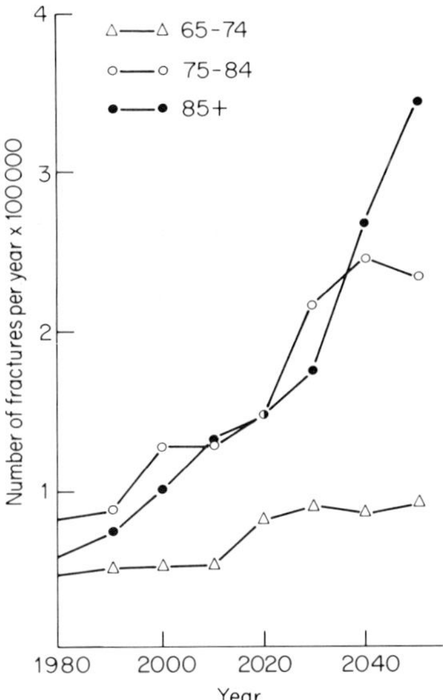

Figure 1.1 Projected number of hip fractures annually in the United States by age: 1980–2050. Source: NCHS and US Bureau of Census projections. (Reproduced by permission from *Nature*, 1985, **315**: 463–465, Macmillan Journals Ltd © and J. A. Brody.)

syncope of unknown cause. In contrast, the cause of syncope was identified in only 13 of 121 patients hospitalized for an average of nine days (Kapoor *et al.*, 1982a).

A prospective study by Kapoor *et al.* (1983) was designed to study the problem further and to determine the prognosis in patients in the year following the onset of syncope. Of the 204 patients enrolled, the diagnosis was established in 107, and in 103 of these it was made at the initial evaluation. Of the 107, 53 patients had a cardiovascular cause of syncope. Their 12-month mortality was 30 ± 6.7%. This was significantly higher than the 12 ± 4.4% mortality in patients with non-cardiovascular syncope and the 6.4 ± 2.8% mortality in patients with no known cause. The patients with cardiovascular syncope were significantly older and more often had previously diagnosed cardiac risk factors as opposed to the patients with non-cardiovascular syncope or syncope of unknown cause. Overall cumulative mortality in the entire group was 14% and the rate of sudden death was 8%. Of the 106 patients in whom a positive diagnosis was established, the diagnostic methods and their yields are shown in Table 1.1. History taking alone was diagnostic in 50%. Of the 101 patients without an aetiological diagnosis at the start of the study, only four had a precise diagnosis after one year of observation.

Day *et al.* (1982) examined 198 consecutive patients presenting at an emergency room with transient loss of consciousness. They were able to diagnose 172 on the initial assessment and were unsuccessful with 25 of the remaining 26 despite extensive further investigations.

Dermkisan and Lamb (1958) studied 82 persons and 113 syncopal episodes amongst healthy United States Air Force flying personnel. Ages ranged from 18 to 40 years. The most

Table 1.1 Successful diagnostic methods in 106 of 204 patients with syncope. The remainder were undiagnosed after the initial work-up. (Reproduced by permission from Wishwa Kapoor *et al.* and the *New England Journal of Medicine,* 1983, **309**(4): 197–204.)

Study	Number of patients
History and physical	52
Electrocardiography	12
Electrocardiographic monitoring	29
Electrophysiologic studies	3
Cardiac catheterization	7
Cerebral angiography	2
Electroencephalography	1
Total	106*

* In one additional patient a diagnosis of aortic dissection was made at autopsy, seven days after the patient presented with syncope.

common overt fact at the moment of the syncope was a change in posture or pain. Eleven of the 82 had at least one alcoholic drink prior to the syncope, six had been on weight-reduction diets, and others had recently completed exhaustive physical labour and/or were chronically tired. Fifty-five of the 82 were examined by special techniques that provoked a syncopal or near syncopal episode in 16. The provocative techniques were: the use of atropine causing a shift in pacemaker to an atrial focus, carotid sinus massage, breath holding, hyperventilation, or being placed on a tilt table. None had evidence of heart disease.

History

> "The description of the attack is valuable. The patient with simple syncope is pale, with Stokes–Adams attack he looks dead. The quick recovery, usually short duration, and historical details from the patient are not seen with epilepsy. When the patient is recovered from an attack and attempts to get up with the return of the light-headed pre-syncopal feeling, the diagnosis is almost always orthostatic or vasovagal fainting and never a Stokes–Adams attack" (Fisher, 1979).

Many patients who faint have a few jerking movements of the limbs while unconscious. Fainters are also sometimes incontinent of urine while unconscious. The reduced cerebral perfusion of syncope from any cause may stimulate a full epileptic seizure in a suitable individual. The differentiation of fit versus faint is not always easy. The reverse situation, a seizure disorder causing intermittent heart block leading to syncope is described in Chapter 13.

The diagnostic possibilities suggested from various key features in the history are listed at the end of this chapter.

DIAGNOSTIC METHODS

A retrospective study of 121 patients, average age 63 years, hospitalized for syncope of unknown origin over a four-year period revealed the cause of the syncope in only 13. The average hospital stay was nine days and the average cost was $2463 per patient. The yield from various investigative procedures varied. Cardiac monitoring in 67 patients showed diagnostic abnormalities in seven. Thirteen patients underwent electrophysiological studies. Four of these had diagnostically abnormal results and cardiac catheterization in 14 patients made the diagnosis in only three (Kapoor *et al.*, 1982a).

Unhelpful tests were glucose tolerance test, head computed tomography (CT) scan, radionuclide brain scan, lumbar puncture, and skull x-ray. Twenty-six of 67 patients had abnormal EEGs. The significance or application of these to the diagnosis of syncope could not be defined. Gendelman *et al.* (1983) studied 205 syncopal patients. Head CT scanning produced no useful information in patients free from neurological signs and symptoms, but revealed diagnostic information in 8% of patients with signs and/or symptoms. The EEG provided evidence of a previously unknown seizure disorder in none.

A prospective study of 204 patients with syncope was carried out by Kapoor *et al.* (1983). The results were startlingly different from their retrospective study of 1982. In the more recent collection, a cardiovascular cause was established in 53 patients and a non-cardiovascular cause in 54. Ninety-seven patients remained undiagnosed as to cause. It has been suggested by Kapoor *et al.* (1984) that patients with syncope of unknown origin (after a thorough and logical investigation) are younger, have a lower incidence of cardiovascular disease, a more favourable prognosis, and should be considered as an independent clinical group. In 93 of 106 patients with syncope of known cause the primary diagnosis was apparent from the initial history, physical examination, ECG or Holter monitoring (Table 1.1).

Prolonged portable ECG monitoring is an essential part of the evaluation. How long to monitor a patient is not settled and precise diagnostic criteria have yet to be established. Kapoor *et al.* (1984) found a poor correlation between symptoms during monitoring and concurrent ECG findings. Light-headedness or syncope during monitoring occurred in 30–40% of patients (Clark *et al.*, 1980; Kapoor *et al.*, 1982b). These same authors found that a disturbance of rhythm could not be identified during 75% of the symptomatic periods. It has been suggested that monitoring continue until the symptoms occur (Van Durme, 1975). Alternatively, Johannson (1981) indicated that little information was obtained by monitoring beyond 24 hours.

Critchley and Wright (1983) believed ambulatory, 24-hour, Holter ECG monitoring was of value in all patients with a questionable diagnosis and for suspected arrhythmias. Intermittent changes in rhythm are likely to be of pathological importance if accompanied by symptoms, and a cardiac cause may be found for blackouts masquerading as epilepsy or transient ischaemic attacks. Camm and Levy (1983) thought the yield from ambulatory monitoring was low, although the test is cheap, non-invasive, and safe. Gibson and Levy (1982) analysed 1512 cardiogram tapes recorded in an attempt to diagnose an arrhythmic cause of syncope. Fifteen patients suffered syncope while recording; in only seven was an arrhythmia responsible. Kapoor *et al.* (1982b) had a similar low yield of 10% positive diagnoses from ambulatory cardiography. Of the 205 patients studied by Gendelman *et al.* (1983), Holter monitoring for 24 hours uncovered arrhythmias predisposing to syncope in 21% of the whole group. They did not differentiate whether monitoring was more revealing in patients with clinical evidence of heart disease than in those without. On admission, 43 of their patients had a diagnosis of syncope due to cardiac causes; on discharge 55 patients had this diagnosis.

Similarly, Luxon *et al.* (1980) found that 33% of their patients with unexplained syncope had a significant arrhythmia and Jonas *et al.* (1977), who examined 358 patients, reported a frequency of about 20% of their patients with syncope or pre-syncope had significant arrhythmias on Holter monitoring.

Lai and Ziegler (1981) have summarized the topic thus:

> "Interpretation of the clinical relevance of electrocardiographic data requires astute judgment. Apparently benign complex arrhythmias and conduction defects are frequently detected in healthy people but many of the subtler forms of heart block and dysfunction of the sinus node where a cardiac pacemaker would be beneficial to the patient are still underdiagnosed. Given a reasonably high index of suspicion, prolonged electrocardiographic recordings over a minimum period of 72 hours are advisable. Monitoring the electrocardiogram and electroencephalogram may serve to confirm a cardiac cause for an apparent cerebral event or an arrhythmia provoked by an apneic episode in sleep or at the onset of a seizure."

Intracardiac electrophysiological studies can be revealing with a potentially high yield in the diagnosis and management of patients with syncope. The negative factors are that some of the reasons for assigning a cause for syncope based on these studies are debatable. There are reliable data concerning sustained unimorphic ventricular tachycardias, markedly prolonged HV (His bundle–ventricle) interval (more than 80 msec), and prolonged sinus node recovery time in patients with unexplained syncope. However, the significance of non-sustained polymorphic ventricular tachycardia, mildly prolonged HV interval, or sinus node recovery time, and induction of supraventricular tachycardia is not clear. In addition, these studies are invasive, done only in specialized centres, are expensive, and relatively dangerous.

PHYSICAL ASSESSMENT

In addition to a cardiovascular assessment, a complete neurological examination must be done. Abnormal neurological signs may reveal evidence of a cerebral lesion and a correct diagnosis of epilepsy. Syringobulbia and syringomyelia and other disorders at the atlanto–occipital junction, Arnold–Chiari malformation, etc. may be associated with syncope on changing head posture, coughing, or straining. Measurement of erect and supine blood pressure indicating orthostatic hypotension as well as massage of the carotid sinus which may reveal a true carotid sinus syndrome, an atrioventricular conduction defect or sino-atrial disorder, should be routine. These should be hospital procedures with simultaneous cardiogram, EEG, and blood-pressure recordings. They are considered in detail in later chapters.

If the possibility of hypovolaemia, orthostatic hypotension, or endocrine dysfunction is evident, further laboratory tests are required. A chest x-ray and standard 12-lead ECG are obligatory. Any defect of atrio-ventricular conduction or evidence of inferior wall myocardial infarction should raise the possibility of Stokes–Adams attacks and anterior myocardial infarction, pre-excitation syndromes. These are characterized by a short PR interval and abnormal QRS complex or prolonged QT interval, and should warn of the possibility of life-threatening tachyarrhythmias. Echocardiography is useful in the diagnosis of hypertrophic cardiomyopathy, atrial myxoma, mitral-valve prolapse, or amyloid heart disease (Critchley and Wright, 1983).

Critchley and Wright (1983) believed that exercise testing and trials of cardiac pacing are often unhelpful. Further, they stated that electrophysiological studies are risky and of doubtful value and quote DiMarco *et al.* (1981) as support. Camm and Levy (1983) disagree strongly and have stated

> "thus in recurrent syncope . . . both ambulatory electrocardiographic monitoring (low yield but relatively cheap and non-invasive) and electrophysiological studies (expensive and invasive but potentially high yield) must be considered when clinical circumstances demand an accurate diagnosis".

Gibson and Levy (1982) and Kapoor *et al.* (1982b) had a low yield of positive diagnoses from ambulatory recording of patients with syncope (see above). In contrast, electrophysiological testing was diagnostic in 94 of 149 (63%) patients with recurrent syncope. Most of them had normal resting, ambulatory and stress cardiograms and neurological investigations. Appropriate therapy was instituted and 87% of the diagnosed patients were then symptom free (Brandenburg *et al.*, 1981; DiMarco *et al.*, 1981; Hess *et al.*, 1982).

Hess *et al.* (1982) and DiMarco *et al.* (1981) found an unexpectedly high (34–36%) incidence of unsuspected ventricular tachycardias which were effectively treated with antiarrhythmic drugs chosen from information gained by electrophysiological assessment.

Gulamhusein *et al.* (1982) reported some opposing views and indicated the limitations of electrophysiological study in assessing unexplained syncope. They studied 34 patients with unexplained syncope or pre-syncope. The entire group had normal ECGs, clinical examinations, ambulatory ECG recordings and treadmill testing. The electrophysiological studies were diagnostic in 11% of the group, were abnormal but not diagnostic in 5%, and were normal in the remainder. During an average follow-up of 15 months, 47% of the group had no further episodes in the absence of intervention and the diagnosis became evident in another 12%. In seven patients permanent pacing was instituted empirically with relief of the syncope.

They concluded that the diagnostic yield of electrophysiological testing was **low** in a patient population that had no ECG abnormalities or clinical evidence of cardiac disease. Empirical pacing in patients with persistent symptoms (after electrophysiological testing) appeared to be beneficial. However, there was a high incidence of spontaneous remission in this group as well.

The consensus seems to be that a meticulous history, physical examination and an ECG are the cornerstones of evaluation. When a cause is not evident, 24-hour ECG monitoring is the next step and possibly an additional 24 hours of monitoring in patients in whom an arrhythmia is suspected but not diagnosed.

Invasive electrophysiological studies should be reserved for patients with frequent recurrent symptoms but without known structural heart disease, in whom appropriate clinical evaluation and monitoring have not shown the cause of syncope.

Kapoor *et al.* (1986) evaluated 210 elderly patients (mean age 71) and 190 younger patients (mean age 39), all with syncope. A cardiovascular explanation for the fainting was obtained in 33% of the former group and in 16.8% of the latter. Non-cardiovascular or cause unknown was the final diagnosis in 26% and 38%, respectively in the elderly group, while the equivalent figures for the younger group were 37% and 45%.

ECG monitoring established the diagnosis in 17% of the elderly but in only 8% of the

Table 1.2 Possible syncopal mechanisms related to the clinical setting

If syncope usually/always occurs in the following situations:	Probability of the following diagnosis or mechanisms:
• With arm exercise	Subclavian steal
• With head rotation or extension	Atlanto–occipital joint disease Syringomyelia/bulbia Arnold–Chiari malformation Atheroma vertebrobasilar vessels Carotid sinus syndrome
• With trunk movement, i.e. from sitting to lying, or bending at the waist, or turning over in bed	Atrial myxoma or thrombus and/or cardiac rhythm/conduction defect—sinus node or atrioventricular
• Carotid sinus compression, tumour, or massage, or head rotation	Cardiac rhythm/conduction defect—sinus node or atrioventricular Peripheral vasodepressor response with or without cardiac rhythm/conduction defect—sinus node or atrioventricular
• Pressure on, examination of, or instrumentation of, eye, ear, throat, nose, vagina, bladder, rectum—while or after micturition, while defaecating, during sexual intercourse	Cardiac rhythm/conduction defect—sinus node or atrioventricular Peripheral vasodepressor response with or without cardiac rhythm/conduction defect—sinus node or atrioventricular
• A deaf child, on effort or with emotional distress (and positive family history)	Prolonged QT syndrome of Lange–Nielsen
• A non-deaf infant, on effort or with emotional distress (and positive family history)	Prolonged QT syndrome of Romano–Ward
• Adult on effort	Aortic stenosis–congenital or acquired Idiopathic hypertrophic subaortic stenosis Coronary artery disease (may faint before chest pain) Mitral stenosis Myocarditis
• Young adult, usually female, on effort	Pulmonary hypertension
• With postural change from sitting to lying to standing:	Thrombus in atrium Myxoma in atrium
• On standing:	
– frequently in middle-aged or elderly,	Autonomic neuropathy. In any situation where cerebral blood flow is already compromised, i.e. bilateral carotid artery occlusion, or severe stenosis; increased intracranial pressure
– single episode after prolonged bed-rest, debilitating illness, hunger, dehydration	Temporary autonomic nervous system retardation
– single episode, prolonged standing at attention	Vasovagal
– hot weather, after meals, after alcohol	Autonomic neuropathy
• In a well-trained athlete; after exhausting physical exercise	Peripheral vasodepressor response plus bradyarrhythmia

Table 1.2 *continued*

If syncope usually/always occurs in the following situations:	Probability of the following diagnosis or mechanisms:
• At the sight, sound, or smell of something unpleasant, following sudden unexpected pain	Vasovagal response—peripheral vasodepressor plus cardiac dysrhythmia
• With glossopharyngeal neuralgia or trigeminal neuralgia	Cardiac dysrhythmia plus possible peripheral vasodepressor
• With swallowing hot, cold, or room temperature solids or liquids	Oesophageal disease plus cardiac dysrhythmia and peripheral vasodepressor response
• While coughing	Raised intrathoracic pressure, reduced cardiac filling and therefore output; raised intracranial pressure and reduced cerebral blood flow—A–V heart block, atlanto–occipital junction abnormality
• In association with transient cerebral ischemic attacks and/or systemic emboli	Atrial myxoma Mitral valve prolapse Sick sinus syndrome Other disorders of cardiac rhythm
• In a weightlifter—while lifting	Valsalva manoeuver plus the effect of coming out of a full knee bend
• Sudden abrupt syncope—no prodrome	Cardiac conduction disorder
• Slow onset syncope—on return of consciousness and assuming upright position, symptoms return	Vasovagal disorder
• Extended syncope (15–30 min), or brief syncope, focal neurological episodes, epileptic seizures with breathlessness and chest discomfort	Sick sinus syndrome
• Syncope with flushing, palpitation, and itching	Mastocytosis

young. Syncope resulted in trauma to about one-third of both groups and the two-year overall mortality was 26.9% in the elderly and 8.3% in the young. When the young and old had a cardiovascular diagnosis, the overall mortality and incidence of sudden death was the same. However, in the elderly with a diagnosis of non-cardiovascular disease or unknown cause, the mortality and incidence of sudden death were higher. A cardiovascular cause of syncope was a very strong risk factor.

In the elderly group with a cardiovascular aetiology, the most common diagnosis was ventricular tachycardia (33 patients). Sick sinus syndrome was the second most common (12 patients). Complete heart block was present in five, aortic stenosis in eight and myocardial infarction in four patients. Orthostatic hypotension was the most common non-cardiovascular cause (18 patients) and syncope related to coughing, micturition or defaecation, was the second most common (15 patients).

In summary, this study reveals that syncope in younger patients is a premonitoring symptom of sudden death only when a cardiovascular cause is documented. In contrast, elderly patients with syncope have a poor prognosis regardless of the diagnosis and those with a cardiovascular cause have an even worse prognosis. Some useful clinical clues to the cause of syncope are listed in Table 1.2.

REFERENCES

Brody JA (1984) Facts, projections, and gaps concerning data on ageing. *Public Health Reports* **99**: 468–475.

Brody JA (1985) Prospects for an ageing population. *Nature* **315**: 463–466.

Brandenburg RO, Holmes DR and Hartzler GD (1981) The electrophysiologic assessment of patients with syncope. *American Journal of Cardiology* **47**: 433.

Camm AJ and Levy AM (1983) Evaluation of syncope. *British Medical Journal* **286**: 895 (letter).

Clark PI, Glasser SP and Spoto E (1980) Arrhythmias detected by ambulatory monitoring: lack of correlation with symptoms of dizziness and syncope. *Chest* **6**: 722–725.

Critchley EMR and Wright JS (1983) Evaluation of syncope. *British Medical Journal* **286**: 500–501.

Day SC, Cook EF, Funkenstein H and Goldman L (1982) Evaluation and outcome of emergency room patients with transient loss of consciousness. *American Journal of Medicine* **73**: 15–23.

Dermkisan G and Lamb LE (1958) Syncope in a population of healthy young adults. *Journal of the American Medical Association* **168**(9): 1200–1207.

DiMarco JP, Garan H, Harthorne JW and Ruskin JN (1981) Intracardiac electrophysiologic techniques in recurrent syncope of unknown cause. *Annals of Internal Medicine* **95**: 542–548.

Fisher CM (1979) Syncope of obscure nature. *Canadian Journal of Neurological Sciences* **6**(1): 7–20.

Friedberg CK (1973) Fainting: causes and cures. *Medical Times* **101**(7): 41–55.

Gendelman HE, Linzer M, Gabelman M, Smaller S and Scheuer J (1983) Syncope in a general hospital patient population. *New York State Journal of Medicine* Nov.–Dec. (11–12): 1161–1165.

Gibson TC and Levy AM (1982) Ambulatory EKG monitoring as a screening test in patients with syncope. *Circulation* **66**: 11–73.

Gulamhusein S, Naccarelli GV, Ko T, Prystowsky EN, Barnett HJM, Heger JJ and Klein GJ (1982) Value and limitations of clinical electrophysiologic study in assessment of patients with unexplained syncope. *The American Journal of Medicine* **73**: 700–705.

Harvey WP (1982) *Current Problems in Cardiology*, Vol. 7, No. 7, pp. 1-40. Chicago: Year Book Medical Publishers.

Hess DS, Morady F and Scheinman MM (1982) Electrophysiologic testing in the evaluation of patients with syncope of undetermined origin. *American Journal of Cardiology* **50**: 1309–1315.

Johannson BW (1981) Evaluation of alteration of consciousness and palpitations. In *Ambulatory Electrocardiographic Recording* (eds NK Wenger, MB Mock and I Ringvest) pp. 321–330. Chicago: Year Book Medical Publishers.

Jonas S, Klein I and Dimant J (1977) Importance of Holter monitoring in patients with periodic cerebral symptoms. *Annals of Neurology* **1**: 470–474.

Kapoor WN, Karpf M, Maher Y, Miller RA and Levey GS (1982a) Syncope of unknown origin: the need for a more cost effective approach to its diagnostic evaluation. *Journal of the American Medical Association* **247**: 2687–2691.

Kapoor W, Peterson J and Karpf M (1982b) Ambulatory monitoring in patients with syncope: lack of correlation between symptoms and simultaneous cardiographic findings. *Clinical Research* **30**: 196A (abstract).

Kapoor WN, Karpf M, Wieand S, Peterson JR and Levey GS (1983) A prospective evaluation and follow-up of patients with syncope. *New England Journal of Medicine* **309**(4): 197–204.

Kapoor W, Karpf M and Levey GS (1984) Issues in evaluating patients with syncope. *Annals of Internal Medicine* **100**(5): 755–757.

Kapoor W, Snustad D, Peterson J, Wieand HS, Cha R and Karpf M (1986) Syncope in the elderly. *American Journal of Medicine* **80**(3): 419–428.

Lai C-W and Ziegler DK (1981) Syncope problem solved by continuous ambulatory simultaneous EEG/ECG recording. *Neurology (New York)* **31**: 1152–1154.

Luxon LM, Crowther A, Harrison MJ *et al.* (1980) Controlled study of 24 hour ambulatory electrocardiographic monitoring in patients with transient neurologic symptoms. *Journal of Neurology, Neurosurgery, and Psychiatry* **43**: 37–41.

Savage DD, Corwin L, McGee DL, Kannell WB and Wolf PA (1985) Epidemiologic features of isolated syncope: The Framingham Study. *Stroke* **16**(4): 626–629.

Van Durme JP (1975) Tachyarrhythmias and transient cerebral ischemic attacks. *American Heart Journal* **89**: 538–540.

Wayne HH (1961) Syncope: physiological considerations and an analysis of the clinical characteristics in 510 patients. *American Journal of Medicine* **30**: 418–438.

2

Homeostasis

This chapter describes briefly some of the structures and mechanisms that maintain a stable circulatory system. This is a large topic with components in the cerebral cortex, hypothalamus, brainstem, spinal cord, peripheral sensory, motor and autonomic nervous systems. In addition, various humoral agents—catecholamines, amines, peptides, mineral- and glucocorticoids, the enzyme renin, as well as sodium, chloride, potassium, and calcium, and other substances—take part in the regulation of blood pressure, cardiac output and blood volume, and contribute to vasomotor stability.

Monographs and review articles have been written by Natelson (1985), Reid (1983), and Johnson *et al.* (1984). Figure 2.1, reprinted from Natelson (1985), shows some areas of the brain that exhibit control of the heart, parasympathetic and sympathetic structures.

HIGHER CEREBRAL LEVELS

Mental arithmetic, anger, and fear can elevate the blood pressure and pulse, producing neurogenic hypertension and tachycardia. Bad news, the sight, sound, or smell of something unpleasant may decrease peripheral resistance, lower blood pressure, and cause a faint. Biofeedback and relaxation practices can also lower blood pressure. Acute psychological stress may precipitate ventricular fibrillation via the sympathetic autonomic nervous system (Lown *et al.*, 1977). Similar stresses have been implicated in causing coronary artery spasm and myocardial infarction without thrombosis (Maseri *et al.*, 1978).

There is convincing evidence that brain disease can cause or at least set the stage for heart disease (Lown and DeSilva, 1978). Syncope initiated by a shock or fright clearly is dependent on perception, imagination, and awareness that only the fully functional and integrated higher cerebral levels can provide.

The Hypothalamus

The paraventricular nucleus (PVN) of the hypothalamus is anatomically and physiologically connected to a number of brain-stem cell groups including the locus ceruleus, raphe nuclei, and intermediolateral (IML) grey area of the spinal cord (Fig. 2.1). The latter gives rise to sympathetic preganglionic fibres. The PVN also connects with the norepinephrine-containing

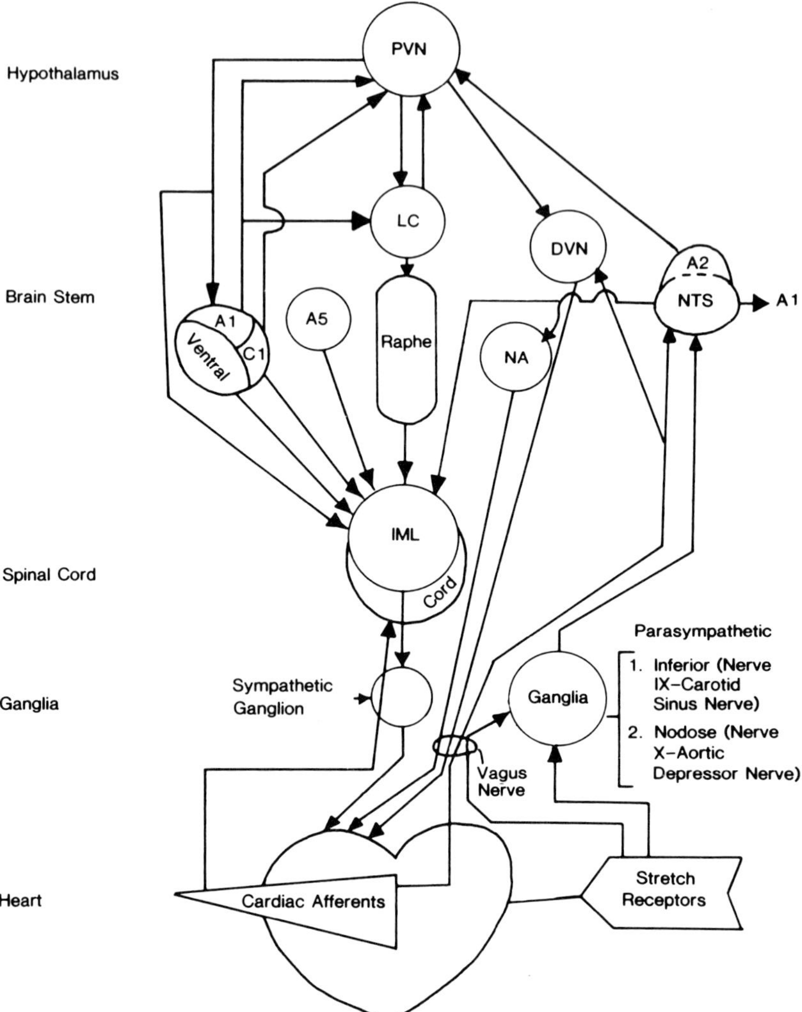

Figure 2.1 Schematic drawing of central and peripheral nervous system/cardiac connections, efferent and afferent with intermediate structures. A1 represents norepinephrine-containing neurones found in the caudal ventrolateral medulla and the locus ceruleus. C1 represents epinephrine-containing neurones in the rostral ventral medulla, A5 the norepinephrine-containing neurones in the ventral pons. Key: PVN = paraventricular nucleus, LC = locus ceruleus, DVN = dorsal nucleus of vagus, NTS = nucleus of tractus solitorius, NA = nucleus ambiguous, IML = intermediolateral grey area. (Reprinted with permission of B. H. Natelson and *Archives of Neurology*, 1985, **42**: 178–183.)

caudal ventrolateral neurones of the medulla as well as the epinephrine-containing neurones in the rostral ventral medulla.

Electrical stimulation of the anterior hypothalamus causes a drop in blood pressure, slow pulse, and blunts the baroreflex responses (Hilton, 1963; McAllen, 1976). Destruction of these areas decreases the baroreflexes.

Nucleus Tractus Solitarius (NTS)

This medullary structure, as well as the paramedian reticular nucleus, receives from the heart and major vessels afferent impulses arising in stretch receptors (baroreceptors) and chemoreceptors. Afferent pathways include the carotid sinus, glossopharyngeal, and vagus nerves and the spinal cord. The NTS has both afferent and efferent connections with the dorsal and ambiguous nuclei of the vagus.

These parasympathetic nuclei also send fibres to the IML grey column. This in turn receives fibres from numerous higher structures including the nucleus tractus solitarius, the anterior hypothalamic nuclei, nuclei of the ventral and lateral medulla, and the raphe nuclei.

Bilateral destruction of the NTS abolishes baroreflexes; a sharp rise in blood pressure occurs which can be prevented with α-adrenoreceptor antagonists.

Efferent Pathways

The main parasympathetic efferent system are vagus fibres to the heart, lung and upper gastrointestinal tract. There is a sacral parasympathetic outflow to pelvic organs.

The cell bodies in the IML grey column in the thoracic and upper lumbar cord give rise to sympathetic efferent preganglionic fibres. These synapse in the sympathetic ganglia and the postsynaptic neurones widely innervate smooth muscle, heart, kidney, gut and other organs. The preganglionic neurones are cholinergic and the postganglionic neurones adrenergic.

Lateralization

Natelson (1985) has summarized some of the evidence suggesting predominance of right- or left-sided structures in autonomic function.

The feline right cerebral hemisphere (Rosen *et al.*, 1982), right medulla (Henry and Calaresu, 1974), right half of the spinal cord (Faden *et al.*, 1978), and the canine right ventral roots (Norris *et al.*, 1977), right stellate ganglia (Randal and Rohse, 1956), as well as right vagus (Hamlin and Smith, 1968), all appear to be dominant in the control of heart rate. However, left-sided canine structures seem to dominate in the production of rhythm disturbances. Left stellate stimulation is more effective in contributing to ventricular fibrillation (Verrier, 1980). Removal of the left stellate is more protective than removal of the right or both ganglia in the production of ouabain-induced tachycardia and death (Kujime and Natelson, 1984).

The parasympathetic system has similar divisions. The right vagus is the dominant parasympathetic nerve to the sino-atrial node and stimulation can evoke sinus arrest. The atrioventricular node is principally supplied by the left vagus. Stimulation of it can produce AV block (Hageman *et al.*, 1975).

Afferent Pathways and Receptors

The awake brain at its highest level is a superb receptor and may initiate wide changes in cardiovascular responses. This depends entirely on the interpretation and experience of the subject.

At the subconscious level, mechano-receptors usually called baroreceptors are present in the proximal aorta, carotid sinus (high-pressure receptors), great veins, pulmonary arteries and the atria (low-pressure receptors). The former respond to change in vessel length and are stimulated by steady and episodic changes. These sensors probably cease discharging altogether when the mean blood pressure drops below 50 mmHg. They are most active with rapidly rising blood pressure and a wide pulse pressure. Impulses are transmitted to the medulla via the carotid sinus and glossopharyngeal nerves. At the medulla there is both inhibitory reduction of pressor area output and stimulation of the depressor area. Simultaneously, the cardiac excitatory centre is inhibited with increased vagal influence on the heart. The net result is a drop in cardiac output and dilatation of peripheral resistance vessels and a lower blood pressure.

There are two types of receptors in the atria, one for pressure, and one for volume. They are most effectively stimulated by a full or over-filled atrium, their afferent nerve is the vagus and the destination of their impulses is the medulla, hypothalamus and supra-optic area. Their function is inhibitory. Stimulation of these receptors restrains the secretion of vasopressin (antidiuretic hormone, ADH) thereby limiting extracellular fluid volume. A reduction in volume (haemorrhage) would enhance vasopressin secretion, which in turn would lead to increased renal re-absorption of water and restore volume towards normal.

Chemoreceptors within the carotid and aortic bodies respond to diminished pH and arterial oxygen tension. Stimulation results in increased ventilation. Cardiovascular changes via these receptors are somewhat less than the direct effect of chemical changes on the brainstem cardiovascular centres. Whether the cardiovascular stimulation is via peripheral receptors or direct on medullary centres, the net effect is a sympathetic stimulation to the heart and circulation.

Cardiovascular Centres

These areas of the medulla, vasoconstrictor and vasodilator, cardio-inhibitory and cardio-excitatory, are justifiably separated on a physiological basis. Their afferent, efferent and internuncial connections as well as what stimulates and inhibits them will not be discussed here. There are many fine descriptions suitable for clinical purposes (see Little, 1985).

CATECHOLAMINES AND PERIPHERAL AUTONOMIC NERVES

The peripheral autonomic system is mentioned briefly in the chapters on the various types of syncope. The key element in peripheral vascular resistance is the tone, or absence of tone, in the pre-capillary muscle sphincter. A host of substances augment or inhibit this structure including blood pressure, epinephrine, norepinephrine, acetylcholine, oxygen, carbon dioxide tension, and pH of the blood and other substances.

Dilator and constrictor vasomotor fibres are rich in some organs and sparse in others. Muscle and gut have more vasoconstrictor fibres than heart or brain and skin has the most of any organ. However, the response to sympathetic stimulation is dependent on more than just the richness of the sympathetic nerve supply.

Norepinephrine (NE) is the vasoconstrictor substance and the dilator is acetylcholine and other less well-understood substances. Epinephrine (E) is both a constrictor and dilator depending on which of the β-receptors it activates. Resting levels of plasma NE and E can be an index of prevailing sympathetic nervous system activity (Lake *et al.*, 1976). In 16 quadraplegic subjects with complete cord lesions, blood pressure, plasma NE and E were significantly lower than in controls. Stimulation of bladder and muscle raised the blood pressure and the plasma catecholamine levels but the latter never exceeded the resting level of normal subjects (Mathias *et al.*, 1976).

The relative contribution to peripheral resistance of various vascular beds can be estimated from A–V differences in plasma NE across the bed and the proportion of cardiac output distributed to it (Goldstein, 1983).

Measurement of major NE metabolites in the urine is helpful in differentiating the various types of sympathetic neuronal dysfunction (Kopin *et al.*, 1983). Polinsky *et al.* (1984) have measured the essential brain metabolite of NE in CSF and plasma as a guide in separating multiple system atrophy from idiopathic orthostatic hypotension. The levels of NE and E in plasma and their kinetics are discussed further in the chapter on autonomic failure (see Chapter 6).

The regulation and balance between vascular tone and cardiac activity maintains the stability of the cardiovascular system. There are both inhibitory and excitatory influences on vascular tone which results in the redistribution of cardiac output. Local needs related to function and the metabolic state also determine the proportion of the blood volume to any one area.

The skeletal muscle vascular bed is an essential organ in maintaining cardiovascular stability via vasomotor reflexes. The pre- and post-capillary resistance vessels and the capacitance vessels (mostly the large veins) are of the greatest importance. The resistance function is involved in the regulation of arterial blood pressure and the ratio of pre- to post-capillary resistance determines hydrostatic pressure and fluid filtration exchange. The smooth-muscle pre-capillary sphincters can reduce the size of the capillary surface available for normal exchange. Transcapillary fluid movement determines plasma volume and changes in regional blood volume affect return and therefore cardiac filling.

The vasoconstrictor fibres of the intestine can make a large volume of blood available to circulatory beds as the constrictor effects will persist as long as sympathetic stimulation is maintained. Vasoconstriction of skin vessels is mostly concerned with thermoregulation and of little consequence in terms of volume of blood sequestered or made available, as compared to muscle and gut.

REFERENCES

Faden AI, Jacobs T and Woods M (1978) Cardio-accelatory sites in the zona intermedia of the cat spinal cord. *Experimental Neurology* **61**: 301–310.

Goldstein DS, McCarty R, Polinsky RJ and Kopin IJ (1983) Relationship between plasma norepinephrine and sympathetic neural activity. *Hypertension* **5**(4): 552–559.

Hageman GR, Randall WC and Armour JA (1975) Direct and reflex cardiac bradydysrhythmias from small vagal nerve stimulations. *American Heart Journal* **89**: 338–348.

Hamlin RL and Smith CR (1968) Effects of vagal stimulation on S–A and A–V nodes. *American Journal of Physiology* **215**: 560–568.

Henry JL and Calaresu FR (1974) Excitatory and inhibitory inputs from medullary nuclei projecting to spinal cardio-accelatory neurons in the cat. *Experiments in Brain Research* **20**: 485–504.

Hilton SM (1963) Inhibition of baroreceptor reflexes on hypothalamic stimulation. *Journal of Physiology (London)* **165**: 56–57.

Johnson RH, Lambie DG and Spalding JMK (1984) Neurocardiology—The interrelationship between dysfunction in the nervous and cardiovascular systems. In *Major Problems in Neurology*, Vol 13 (ed. Sir John Walton). Eastbourne: W. B. Saunders.

Kopin IJ, Polinsky RJ, Oliver JA, Oddershede IR and Ebert MH (1983) Urinary catecholamine metabolites distinguish different types of sympathetic neuronal dysfunction in patients with orthostatic hypotension. *Journal of Clinical Endocrinology and Metabolism* **57**(3): 632–657.

Kujime K and Natelson BH (1984) Effects of stellectomy on cardiac rhythm disturbance induced by ouabain in guinea pigs. *Journal of Pharmacology and Experimental Therapeutics* **229**: 113–117.

Lake CR, Ziegler MG and Kopin IJ (1976) Use of plasma norepinephrine for evaluation of sympathetic neuronal function in man. *Life Science* **18**: 1315–1326.

Little RC (1985) *Physiology of the Heart and Circulation*, 3rd Edition. Chicago: Year Book Medical Publishers.

Lown B and DeSilva RA (1978) Roles of phychologic stress and autonomic nervous system changes in provocation of ventricular premature complexes. *American Journal of Cardiology* **41**: 979–985.

Lown B, Verrier RL and Rabinowitz SH (1977) Neural and psychologic mechanisms and the problem of sudden cardiac death. *American Journal of Cardiology* **39**: 890–902.

Maseri A, L'Abbate A, Baroldi G *et al.* (1978) Coronary vasospasm as a possible cause of myocardial infarction. *New England Journal of Medicine* **299**: 1271–1277.

Mathias CJ, Christensen NJ, Corbett JL, Frankel HL and Spalding JMK (1976) Plasma catecholamines during paroxysmal neurogenic hypertension in quadriplegic man. *Circulation Research* **39**: 204–208.

McAllen RM (1976) Inhibition of the baroreceptor input to the medulla by stimulation of the hypothalamic defence area. *Journal of Physiology (London)* **257**: 45.

Natelson BH (1985) Neurocardiology—an interdisciplinary area for the 80s. *Archives of Neurology* **42**: 178–184.

Norris JE, Foreman RD and Wurster RD (1977) Responses of canine endocardium to stimulation of the upper thoracic roots. *American Journal of Physiology* **233**: H655–659.

Polinsky RJ, Jimerson DC and Kopin IJ (1984) Chronic autonomic failure, CSF, and plasma 3-methoxy-4-hydroxyphenylglycol. *Neurology (Cleveland)* **34**(7): 979–983.

Randal WC and Rohse WG (1956) The augmentor action of the sympathetic cardiac nerves. *Circulation Research* **4**: 470–477.

Reid JL (1983) Central and peripheral autonomic control mechanisms. In *Autonomic Failure* (ed. Sir Roger Bannister) pp. 17–35. Oxford: Oxford University Press.

Rosen AD, Gur RC, Sussman N *et al.* (1982) Hemispheric asymmetry in the control of heart rate. *Society for Neurosciences Abstracts* **8**: 917.

Verrier RL (1980) Neural factors and ventricular electrical instability. In *Sudden Death* (eds VHE Kulbertus and HJJ Wellens) pp. 137–155. The Hague: Martinus Nijhoff.

3

Vasovagal-Vasodepressor Fainting

This is the common faint. Lewis (1932) proposed the title 'vasovagal' for this syndrome and observed that the hypotension and bradycardia were not equally important in syncope. The bradycardia could be abolished by atropine without preventing the attack, and Lewis suggested that peripheral vasodilatation mediated by nervous influences was an important mechanism. He was right.

Nevertheless, heart slowing and irregularity can be important. It is vagal-mediated. The main cause of the fall of blood pressure is independent of the vagus and lies in the blood vessels. Atropine will raise the pulse rate up to and beyond normal levels during the attack leaving the blood pressure below normal and the patient still pale and unconscious. Attacks have been recorded in which the blood pressure fell with no change in pulse. Thus, Lewis concluded that the principal cause of syncope was vasomotor and not vagal. Lewis thought that vasovagal syncope or common syncope could be brought on by fatigue, fasting, confinement to an overheated, overcrowded room, was more common in the young, and more likely to occur in people who were out of condition or in poor health. The stimulus provoking an attack could often be named.

The common situations which may give rise to a vasovagal faint are:

- Unpleasant sights, sounds or smells
- Sudden unexpected pain
- Sustained upright posture
- Standing quickly after a lengthy period of bed-rest
- Standing quickly after a lengthy period of squatting in a full knee bend
- Hypoxia, heat, hunger, dehydration, and prior alcohol excess, *de novo* or compounding any of the others
- Blood loss—although there is an obvious uniqueness to this, the haemodynamic mechanisms have much in common with vasovagal syncope of other origins
- Spinal anaesthetic

CLINICAL FEATURES

Most people have fainted once, or seen someone faint. In the vasovagal faint, the symptoms progress rather slowly taking up to five minutes or longer before consciousness is lost. The timing is an important differential point as cardiac syncope is often instantaneous.

Patients report some or all of the following: a sensation of warmth, a dry mouth and a desire for more air or fresh air or a drink of water. This is accompanied by or quickly followed by epigastric distress, belching, abdominal cramps, and a desire to have a bowel movement. Some patients have deep sighing respirations, yawning, hyperventilation, and blurred vision as late components of the faint and at this point the patient is pale, sweaty with mydriasis, and becomes unconscious. There may be limb and trunk rigidity, a few coarse jerks of the limbs, or a full epileptic seizure.

Following recovery, the patient is nauseated, tremulous, often has a headache, and a desire to remain recumbent. A diuresis often occurs. The pallor persists after the blood pressure has returned to presyncopal levels.

OCCASIONAL OR BENIGN ORTHOSTATIC FAINTING

Patients with autonomic failure have orthostatic fainting as a major early and, for a time, only symptom. There is another group without autonomic failure who also faint on prolonged standing but only occasionally.

The military and police are aware of this and recognize some members of their forces who are known to faint if kept at attention too long. The truth is that all will faint eventually if kept standing and standing still.

The mechanisms protecting us from fainting in this position are complex and usually efficient. They are more stable in some than others and are more effective some days than others, and become less proficient with fatigue, hunger, recovery from illness, alcohol excess, and a host of common medications. The fainting on short or prolonged quiet standing was also designated as vasovagal by Lewis (1932).

Intramuscular, Subcutaneous and Venous Pressures

Mayerson and Toth (1939) and Mayerson *et al.* (1939) suggested that orthostatic syncope was probably due to diminished venous return from excessive pooling in capillaries and veins of the dependent parts. This is only part of the answer.

Mayerson and Burch (1939) investigated the role of muscle tone in postural syncope. They used seven normal adult males—three of whom never fainted in the upright position while two always did. One fainted only on some occasions. The seventh subject fainted early and consistently. He could not tolerate the upright position beyond 6 min.

A tilt table was used which supported the subject in the upright position with the weight on the buttocks and across the iliac crests. All weight bearing and movement by the legs was eliminated. In those who fainted, signs of syncope were evident within the first few minutes and collapse occurred within 20 min.

Venous pressure in the dorsum of the left foot and in the antecubital vein of the right arm was measured (Burch and Sodeman, 1937, 1939). Subcutaneous pressure was measured in the dorsum of the right foot and in the right calf superficial to the gastrocnemius muscle (Burch and Sodeman, 1937). Intramuscular pressure was measured in the right gastrocnemius and right biceps by a modification of the method described by Henderson *et al.* (1936).

In all cases, upright tilting was followed by an immediate rise in venous, subcutaneous and intramuscular pressures. These were maintained with minor fluctuations for the duration of the tilt. There was no difference in the initial pressure changes in the fainting and non-fainting subjects.

The intramuscular pressure changes, however, differed in the two types of experiment. Where signs of syncope appeared during the experiment the intramuscular pressure curve usually followed those of subcutaneous and venous pressures. When no fainting or pre-fainting symptoms were experienced, the intramuscular pressure showed a *secondary* rise during the subsequent 10–15 min which in every case exceeded the initial rise. *In no case did the maximum values found in the fainting group approach the lowest values found during the tilting period where signs of syncope were not evident.* They measured venous pressure from the dorsum of the foot (with the patient upright) using the fourth intercostal space as the zero pressure level of the right atrium. In no experiment did the venous pressure ever fall below hydrostatic pressure as measured to this reference point. When syncope did not develop, venous pressure in the foot veins exceeded the hydrostatic level by 10–17 cmH_2O. In the fainting experiments, however, the pressure was always within 1–2 cmH_2O of the hydrostatic pressure just before collapse was imminent.

Syncope could be prevented in the fainters by actively increasing their intramuscular pressure. This was done by having the subjects stand on their toes on a support at the lower edge of the tilt table. As long as they did this and kept the intramuscular pressure high no signs of syncope were noted. When the subject was allowed to stand flat on his heels, pressure fell rapidly and he complained of dizziness.

Henderson *et al.* (1936) suggested that intramuscular pressure varied with muscle tone, while Wells *et al.* (1938) believed that intramuscular pressure was determined by the tightness of the overlying fascia, the amount of extravascular fluid, and the degree of filling of the vessels.

The relationship of venous, subcutaneous, and intramuscular pressures in the fainting and non-fainting subjects of Mayerson and Burch (1939) suggests the following:

1. There is an immediate increase in subcutaneous and intramuscular pressure in all subjects when tilted from horizontal to vertical and this appears to be due to venous filling. There is an approximate correlation between the amount of venous pressure increase and the increase in subcutaneous and intramuscular pressure.
2. There is a secondary rise in intramuscular pressure in the non-fainting subjects. This is due to the tonic influence of muscle fibres.
3. The higher intramuscular pressure in the non-fainting subjects is composed of the pressure exerted by extravascular fluid, contents of the blood vessels, plus the component due to the *tone of the muscle fibres*. When tone is low the values for intramuscular pressure approach those for subcutaneous pressure. When tone is absent intramuscular pressure is due to the tightness of the overlying fascia, the extravascular fluid in the muscle, and the degree of filling of blood vessels.

These experiments substantiate the suggestion that muscles support the veins and the absence of muscle tone may impair the venous return resulting in syncope. Upright posture syncope can be prevented by increasing muscle tone by slight movement of the lower extremities.

Standing on the balls of the feet during parade will prevent fainting. Intramuscular pressure of the gastrocnemius has been raised to surprisingly high levels when the weight of the body was held on the toes.

Henderson *et al.* (1936) reported that intramuscular pressure in the gastrocnemius rose from 14 to 31 cmH_2O in the upright position when the tone was high, and signs of syncope or pre-syncope appeared when the tone dropped or remained low. The causes of the differences in the muscle tone are speculative. As one normal person has great variations in tone on separate occasions, an anatomical explanation is unlikely. These variations must be related to functional factors and the observations on one test subject suggested that the psychic state of the individual was of utmost importance.

Hellebrandt *et al.* (1939) made the following observations on intramuscular pressure and tone (see also the section Arteries, below):

> "There is little doubt that as the contraction of motor units become more synchronous the pressures accrue sufficiently to reach values in excess of the normal turgor present in the tissues. It is possible that in short term experiments concerned with relaxation and comfortable standing, the *number* of motor units contracting and the synchronicity of their responses are factors of greater importance in the production of intramuscular pressure than stasis or edema".

VASOVAGAL SYNCOPE WHILE SUPINE

Glick and Yu (1963) examined the vasovagal reaction in the course of cardiac catheterization in 13 patients, all in the supine position and all with heart disease. None became unconscious. They suggested the initial factor in this unique type of vasovagal response was an acute rise in blood pressure and pulse pressure. The resulting baroreceptor stimulation produced excessive generalized inhibition of sympathetic tone resulting in bradycardia, arteriolar dilatation and venodilatation. These accounted for the decrease in cardiac index, fall in total systemic resistance and hypotension.

DERANGEMENTS IN VASOVAGAL REACTION

Heart

Although syncope will still occur when the bradycardia is prevented by atropine, nevertheless, vagus activity can make an important contribution to syncope. Greenfield (1951) induced a typical vasovagal reaction terminating in syncope by presenting repugnant psychic stimuli to a subject and demonstrated periods of asystole of 11 and 7 sec. The same response may occur after sudden severe pain. Carp *et al.* (1961) induced vasodepressor syncope with nitrite and noted that bradycardia or arrhythmia preceded the loss of consciousness. Dermkisan and Lamb (1958) in a study of 83 normal young adults with syncopal episodes were able to produce various cardiac arrhythmias by asking the subject to stop breathing both with and without hyperventilation. The arrhythmias and syncope could be prevented with atropine. There is no doubt that the vagus can play an important contributory role in the pathogenesis of vasovagal responses.

Sarnoff *et al.* (1960) demonstrated that with increasing vagal tone and diminishing sympathetic stimulus, the curve of ventricular function shifted so that a higher filling pressure was required to produce a given stroke output. Also, with the fall in blood pressure, decreased resistance to ventricuar ejection, and reduced ventricular after-load the force of subsequent ventricular contractions is diminished (Imperial *et al.*, 1961).

Arteries

The fall in systemic blood pressure which is part of every vasovagal syncope is due to either a decrease in cardiac index or of arterial tone. Both factors decreased concomitantly in the 10 patients examined by Glick and Yu (1963).

Arterial tone is arteriolar in locale and regulated by the discharges of the sympathetic system. Both pressor and depressor centres of the medulla modulate the tone of the vascular bed and are subject to the afferent impulses from the baroreceptors.

Of increasing interest is the function of the sympathetic vasomotor fibres to skeletal muscles. Stjernberg *et al.* (1986) have measured both spontaneous and induced muscle sympathetic activity in normal and paraplegic men. Microelectrode recordings of impulse activity to muscle in normal subjects have shown that sympathetic outflow contributes to a homeostatic blood-pressure level. The activity consists of bursts of vasoconstrictor impulses temporally related to the cardiac rhythm and most evident during transient blood-pressure reduction. Spontaneous steady-state activity had a mean frequency of 27 bursts per minute. There are reciprocal changes in muscle sympathetic activity related to variations of afferent activity from arterial and cardiopulmonary baroreceptors.

Fagius *et al.* (1985) have measured the sympathetic muscle nerve activity (MSA) in the peroneal nerve, and skin sympathetic activity after bilateral lidocaine blocks of glossopharyngeal and vagus nerves in the neck in two healthy normal subjects. They effectively deafferented the arterial and cardiopulmonary baroreceptors.

Following the block there was a strong increase of muscle nerve sympathetic activity, tachycardia and hypertension. The normal cardiac rhythmicity of MSA disappeared and it became irregular in rhythm and duration. They concluded that the cardiac rhythmicity of MSA is due to baroreceptor influence and that the low level of MSA at rest is due to strong baroreceptor inhibition.

Delius *et al.* (1972) have also demonstrated multi-unit sympathetic activity from muscle nerve fascicles in the median and peroneal nerve of resting, relaxed, human subjects. The impulses had a pulsatile rhythm and bursts of impulses appeared during spontaneously occurring blood-pressure reductions. Temporary blood-pressure elevations were associated with neural silence. These findings confirm sympathetic muscle nerve activity as vasoconstrictor. Their outflow is modulated by strong phasic and tonic inhibitory baroreflex influences. Stimuli such as sudden chest compression, a rapid deep breath, or an electrical shock against the skin, will cause a transient inhibition of the sympathetic discharges lasting a few seconds.

NORMAL VENOUS PRESSURE

In man, the input pressure (to the venous system) is the residual of the systemic blood pressure at the venous end of the capillary bed (7–8 mmHg) and the variable opposing hydrostatic pressure of the column of blood plus the resistance of the venous channels. Doupe *et al.* (1938) studied six normal subjects and measured the pressure in the median basilic vein at the elbow, the great saphenous vein at the ankle, and in the internal jugular bulb with the subjects standing, sitting or lying. The effects of breathing, ice or heat on another limb, or cooling of the limbs, on venous pressure were determined. There is considerable variation (up to 10 mmH_2O) in venous pressure from the same measuring point in different subjects.

While *supine,* the pressure recorded from the median basilic vein was equal to the height of the manubrium sterni above the point of insertion of the needle. Pressures obtained from the long saphenous vein and the internal jugular bulb were also equal to the height of the manubrium sterni above the insertion of the needle. If the arm was elevated so that the point of the needle was above the level of the manubrium sterni, the pressure remaining in the median basilic vein varied, in eight experiments, between 1 and 3 cmH_2O. The degree of elevation above the sternum did not affect this residual pressure and at no time was a negative pressure observed.

In the *erect* posture, the pressure at these three sites was again measured. These measurements showed that the pressure in the venous system is capable of lifting the blood to an adequate level for its return to the heart without the assistance of the pumping action of the muscles. The venous pressure in the foot in the upright position changes with the length of standing time.

Vasodilatation

The effect of vasodilatation on the pressure in the median basilic vein was observed by placing one leg in 45°C water. Peripheral vasodilatation occurred in the finger vessels of the arm under investigation. No change in venous pressure was observed during the dilatation of the peripheral vascular bed.

Vasoconstriction

The effect of transient vasoconstriction on peripheral vessels was observed 50 times in six subjects by applying ice to the skin of part of the body for a few seconds when cutaneous vessels were dilated. This produced a transient fall in venous pressure in both median basilic and long saphenous veins. The decrease in venous pressure was synchronous with the decrease in digit volume and returned to the original level as the decrease in finger volume disappeared.

The fall in venous pressure did not occur if the circulation distal to the needle had been occluded by inflating a sphymomanometer cuff placed around the wrist to a pressure of about 200 mmHg. Similarly, it did not occur in response to stimuli when the peripheral vessels were already constricted.

Similar stimuli produced no change in the pressure in the jugular vein with the subject in either the erect or supine position whether the peripheral blood vessels were in a dilated or constricted state.

Conclusions

Following peripheral vasoconstriction brought about by sensory stimuli, venous pressure temporarily diminished in the arms and legs whether the subject was erect or horizontal, irrespective of the relation of the limb to the body. The results also show that the fall in venous pressure following the sensory stimulus is dependent on alterations in the circulation distal to the needle. Dilatation of the peripheral vascular bed did not change venous pressure.

Venous Pressure and Walking

At the start of walking there is a contraction of gastrocnemius and soleus muscles which compresses the veins of the leg. This raises venous pressure at the ankle and a portion of the blood contained in the veins flows upward out of the leg. The venous valves close preventing backflow and venous pressure in the leg decreases because the leg veins are underfilled.

The decrease in pressure while walking occurs because after the fall in pressure produced by the first step, the calf muscles contract in taking the next step before venous filling is complete and thus additional blood is pumped out of the leg causing a further drop in pressure when the calf muscles relax. This is repeated until as much blood comes into the vein from the capillaries as is pumped out of the leg with each step and the pressure is then stable.

Exercising on a level treadmill at 1.7, 2.6, and 3.3 m.p.h. produces changes similar to those of a single step. The average decrease in pressure irrespective of the speed of walking is approximately 60 mmHg (Pollack and Wood, 1949).

To summarize:

1. The high venous pressure in the legs when upright can have serious consequences if it persists. The muscular contractions associated with walking lower venous pressures in the legs and feet by compression of the leg veins as they travel through the active muscle groups. The pumping aided by the venous valves squeezes the contents towards the heart. When the muscles relax the valves prevent backflow and each deep venous segment fills from the superficial veins and lower deep veins. The venous fluid column between the periphery and the heart is interrupted, and the hydrostatic force exerted on the lower venous segments is reduced, and the venous pressure in the foot is lowered. A single step can be effective in reducing high venous pressure produced by quiet standing.
2. Venous pressure is high enough in the foot or arm of a standing subject to lift a column of blood as high as the atrium without assistance from the pumping action of the leg muscles.
3. This pressure can change as the length of time standing is extended.
4. Constriction of the peripheral vascular bed will cause a fall in venous pressure.
5. Dilatation of the peripheral vascular bed will not change venous pressure.

Increased Venous Capacity

Large varicosities in the saphenous system may be accompanied by dizziness and syncope under the stress of standing. Pharmacological agents that relax smooth-muscle capacitance vessels either directly (nitrites) or indirectly by blocking sympathetic innervation (guanethidine) produce the same response as large varicosities on upright standing. The mechanism is the same as other forms of inadequate venous return. Just prior to syncope in all of these disorders there is a profound bradycardia and fall in peripheral resistance, indicating an overpowering vagal, cholinergic response to the cerebral ischaemia (Hickler and Howe, 1979).

Intrathoracic Venous Pressure

The veins in the thoracic cavity are subject to negative intrapleural pressure. During inspiration the increased negative intrapleural pressure assists venous return to a limited degree. Right ventricular output is also assisted by inspiration. The increased capacity of the pulmonary vascular tree due to inflation of the lungs in inspiration accommodates this output.

The Right Side of the Heart

The activity of the right ventricle increases flow into the right atrium. This is larger during right ventricular systole than diastole. During ventricular contraction, the descent of the A–V junction enlarges the atrium and vena cava. This is helpful in maintaining venous return during tachycardia. In a slow heart, most atrial filling occurs during the long ventricular diastole, but with a rapid heart rate the proportion of atrial filling due to active systolic injection of blood from the veins into the right atrium is greatly increased.

Responses to Initial Rise in Pulse and Blood Pressure

Contraction of veins has little effect on resistance to flow. Ross *et al.* (1961) have established that venous dilatation sequesters blood, reduces venous return and decreases cardiac output. It occurs reflexly, initiated by carotid sinus hypertension.

Glick and Yu (1963) believe that the initial mechanism in the vasovagal response is an acute rise in carotid sinus pressure and pulse pressure. Emotionally-induced faints are also explicable on this basis, as an acute rise in pulse rate and blood pressure are the initial cardiovascular responses in these situations. Graham *et al.* (1961) have recorded this phenomenon and termed it the 'diphasic response in blood donors and venepuncture subjects' who subsequently go on to a vasovagal syncope.

A sudden increase in carotid sinus pressure leads to reflex bradycardia, arteriolar dilatation, lower systemic resistance and blood pressure, and venodilatation and reduced cardiac output. A generalized inhibition of sympathetic tone occurs as well as vagal inhibition of the heart. Lofving (1961) has shown that when sympatho-inhibitory areas of the limbic cortex are stimulated, a response similar to baroreceptor stimulation is elicited plus vagal slowing of the heart.

Why do some people after an acute rise in systemic blood pressure respond with a mild fall in blood pressure during the recovery phase while others go beyond this to an exaggerated, vasovagal reaction? The difference may be the result of the two sympatho-inhibitory influences which play on the vasomotor centres. The baroreceptor mechanisms have obligatory inhibitory impulses and may start the development of the vasovagal response while the limbic centre contribution is, in a sense, 'optional'. The cortical limbic system is concerned with the emotional content of the response and its contribution may be the added factor which precipitates the vasovagal response in a suitable person at an appropriate time.

However, a vasovagal faint can occur without the intitial pulse and blood-pressure elevation, and without the 'optional' psychic contribution from the limbic system. Epstein *et al.* (1968) have demonstrated this. They studied the capacitance and resistance vessels in vasovagal syncope in 10 subjects. Negative pressure below the iliac crest and 80° head-up tilt produced vasovagal reactions in all. The first phase was a gradual fall in arterial pressure during which forearm vascular resistance did not change. The onset of the second phase was marked by an abrupt fall in arterial pressure and heart rate, and a 60% decrease in forearm vascular resistance. Venoconstriction occurred in the forearm and hand veins. Central venous pressure did not change prior to, or during, the reaction and therefore it is unlikely that veno-

Table 3.1 Vasovagal-vasodepressor syncope synopsis

- In vasovagal fainting the bradycardia is not the essential part of the response. If prevented by pretreatment with atropine, the syncope will still occur
- Prolonged standing still causes some otherwise normal people to faint every time and will cause all to faint if the position is held long enough
- Raised intramuscular pressure in the calf helps prevent orthostatic syncope
- Muscle tone and pressure increase immediately on standing and again some minutes after standing in non-fainters (orthostatic). In those who faint, only the initial rise occurs
- In the standing position venous pressure measured from the dorsum of the foot is high enough to fill the right atrium
- The initial tachycardia and hypertension from fear or pain can be followed by bradycardia and hypotension leading to syncope. Whether syncope occurs depends on the strength of this later baroreceptor-induced response and a variable contribution from the limbic system

dilatation occurred in other vascular beds. They concluded that two of the major mechanisms responsible for the hypotension of vasovagal syncope initiated by orthostasis and lower body negative pressure are bradycardia and dilatation of the resistance vessels. In contrast, the venous bed by constricting, tends to maintain filling pressure and cardiac output and thus works in the opposite direction (see Chapter 4).

The important features of vasovagal-vasodepressor syncope are summarized in Table 3.1.

REFERENCES

Burch GE and Sodeman WA (1937) The estimation of subcutaneous tissue pressure by a direct method. *Journal of Clinical Investigation* **16**: 845–850.

Burch GE and Sodeman WA (1939) A direct method for the determination of venous pressure; relationship of tissue pressure to venous pressure. *Journal of Clinical Investigation* **18**: 31–34.

Carp HR, Weissler AM and Heyman A (1961) Vasodepressor syncope. EEG and circulatory changes. *Archives of Neurology and Psychiatry* **5**: 94.

Delius W, Hagbarth K-D, Hongell A and Wallin BG (1972) General characteristics of sympathetic activity in human muscle nerves. *Acta Physiologica Scandinavica* **84**: 65–81.

Dermksian G and Lamb LE (1958) Syncope in a population of healthy young adults. *Journal of the American Medical Association* **168**: 1200.

Doupe J, Krynauw RA and Snodgrass SR (1938) Some factors influencing venous pressure in man. *Journal of Physiology* **92**: 383–400.

Epstein SE (1968) Role of the capacitance and resistance in vessels in vasovagal syncope. *Circulation* **37**: 524–533.

Fagius J, Wallin BG, Sundlof G, Nerhed C and Englesson S (1985) Sympathetic outflow in man after anaesthesia of the glossopharyngeal and vagus nerve. *Brain* **108**: 423–438.

Glick G and Yu PN (1963) Hemodynamic changes during spontaneous vasovagal reactions. *American Journal of Medicine* **34**: 42–51.

Graham DT, Kabler JD and Lunsford L (1961) Vasovagal fainting, a diphasic response. *Psychosomatic Medicine* **23**: 493.

Greenfield ADM (1951) An emotional faint. *Lancet* **1**: 1302.

Hellebrandt FA, Grigler EF and Kelso LEA (1939) Variations in intramuscular pressure during postural and phasic contraction of human muscle. *American Journal of Physiology* **126**: 247–253.

Henderson Y, Oughterson AW, Greenberg LA and Searle CP (1936) Muscle tonus, intramuscular pressure, and the vasopressor mechanism. *American Journal of Physiology* **114**: 261–268.

Hickler RB and Howe JP (1979) Syncope: its etiology, pathophysiology, management. *Primary Cardiology* **4**(3): 46–51.

Imperial ES, Levy MN and Zieske H (1961) Outflow resistance as an independent determinant of cardiac performance. *Circulation Research* **9**: 1148.

Lewis T (1932) Vasovagal syncope and the carotid sinus mechanism. *British Medical Journal* **1**: 873.

Lofving B (1961) Cardiovascular adjustments induced from the rostral singulate gyrus with special reference to sympathetico-inhibitory mechanisms. *Acta Physiologica Scandinavica* **53** (**supplement**): 184.

Mayerson HS and Burch GE (1939) Relationships of tissue (subcutaneous and intramuscular) and venous pressures to syncope induced in man by gravity. *American Journal of Physiology* **128**: 258–269.

Mayerson HS, Sweeney HM and Toth LA (1939) The influence of posture on circulation time. *American Journal of Physiology* **125**: 481–485.

Mayerson HS and Toth LA (1939) The influence of posture on skin and subcutaneous temperatures. *American Journal of Physiology* **125**: 474–480.

Pollock AA and Wood EH (1949) Venous pressure in the saphenous vein of the ankle in man during exercise and changes in posture. *Journal of Applied Physiology* **1**: 649–662.

Ross J, Frahm CJ and Braunwald E (1961) Influence of the carotid baroreceptors and a vasoactive drug on systemic vascular volume and venous distensibility. *Circulation Research* **9**: 75.

Sarnoff SJ, Brockman SK, Gilmore JP, Linden RJ and Mitchell JH (1960) Regulation of ventricular contraction. Influence of cardiac sympathetic vagal nerve stimulation on atrial and ventricular dynamics. *Circulation Research* **8**: 1108.

Stjernberg L, Blumberg H and Wallin G (1986) Sympathetic activity in man after spinal cord injury. *Brain* **109**: 695–715.

Wells HS, Youmans JB and Miller DG (1938) Tissue pressure (intracutaneous, subcutaneous and intramuscular) as related to venous pressure, capillary filtration, and other factors. *Journal of Clinical Investigation* **17**: 489–499.

4

Experimental Syncope

Experimental syncope has been produced using a tilt table, phlebotomy, tourniquets about the thighs, parenteral nitrites and combinations of these methods.

INDUCTION OF SYNCOPE

Nitrites

Nitrites dilate both arterial and venous smooth muscle by an unknown mechanism and in low dosage the effect on veins is greater (Gilman *et al.*, 1980).

High doses given rapidly will lower systolic and diastolic blood pressure and cardiac output and provoke all the common pre-syncopal symptoms and compensatory reflexes.

Organic nitrites dilate venous capacitance and arteriolar resistance vessels. The former decreases venous return to the heart and the latter decreases the force of the left ventricle during systole (Williams *et al.*, 1965). In low doses, in normal subjects, the venous dilatation is greater than the arteriolar, and systemic vascular resistance is unchanged.

Tilt

In man, tilting into the head-up position immediately decreases inferior vena caval flow. Compensation mechanisms begin to restore the venous return but it remains less than in the supine position. Central venous pressure drops by 3–5 mmHg.

When upright, the blood pressure in the carotid sinus and other low-pressure baroreceptors decreases, the heart becomes smaller, cardiac output drops and the pulse increases. Stroke volume decreases by 50% and output by 25%.

The pressure in the dependent veins increases and the filling pressure of the heart drops. Some 500 ml of blood leaves the thorax and accumulates in the lower extremities. As blood pressure drops and peripheral resistance increases, ventricle size diminishes and there is decreased blood flow through skin, skeletal muscles, liver and kidney.

When subjects have been confined to bed for a long period or had a debilitating illness and first assume the upright posture, the muscles of the abdomen and limbs are weak, tone of the nervous mechanisms governing peripheral vessels is lowered and hydrostatic effects are overcome with difficulty. The blood flows into the large abdominal veins and capillaries and the right heart is inadequately filled. The arterial pressure falls and the cerebral blood flow becomes inadequate. The subject turns pale, sweats freely, and feels giddy, nauseated, and may faint (Best and Taylor, 1980).

Syncope Induced with Nitrites and Tilt

Weissler *et al.* (1957) induced vasodepressor syncope by head-up tilt and the use of nitrites. Cardiac output was measured in eight subjects at 60° head-up tilt before and during syncope. Control output was measured 3–10 min after tilting when the subjects were relaxed with stable blood pressure and pulse. The pre-syncopal symptoms occurred at varying and unpredictable intervals **before** the hypotension and bradycardia.

The mean arterial blood pressure for the entire group was 84 mmHg in the control period and 38 mmHg during the faint. Cardiac output during syncope showed a mean fall for the group with an insignificant decrease in cardiac index of 0.4 litre.

Stroke volume changes were variable and showed no consistent trend. During syncope a bradycardia was always observed relative to the usual presyncopal tachycardia. At the time of syncope arterial pCO_2 was consistently decreased by an average of 4.4 vol%.

They concluded that a constant feature of vasodepressor orthostatic syncope was the failure of cardiac output to rise in spite of decreased peripheral resistance. This could be explained by reflex cardiac inhibition or a diminished volume of blood available to the heart. After atropine and a marked tachycardia, the response to a fall in peripheral resistance was no different than in the non-atropinized subjects.

The reduced volume of blood available to the heart was studied by anti-gravity suit inflation, negative pressure breathing and albumin infusion. Each of these either aborted or prevented the hypotensive phase of syncope. Inflation of the anti-gravity suit resulted in termination of the hypotension and a simultaneous increase in cardiac output in spite of the fact that the subjects were maintained upright. This suggests that reduced venous inflow played a significant role in the reduced cardiac output in syncope.

The fall in arterial carbon dioxide was due to the hyperventilation. Hypocapnia results in mild hypotension, increased forearm blood flow, and diminished cerebral blood flow. These add to the circulatory upset of syncope but hyperventilation alone is not the critical component.

In conclusion, syncope produced with a 60° head-up tilt plus sodium nitrite was similar to spontaneous syncope and was marked by a slight drop in cardiac output with an excessive rise in cardiac output during recovery but a failure of cardiac output during the faint to compensate for the major fall in peripheral resistance. The major circulatory event of vasodepressor syncope appeared to be widespread loss of peripheral resistance while the heart was unable to compensate with increased output and this was due to limited venous inflow (Table 4.1).

Weiss *et al.* (1937) also studied normal subjects with syncope induced by nitrites and head-up tilt. The changes preceding any symptoms of syncope were tachycardia and reduced pulse pressure (almost entirely due to a reduction of systolic pressure). A fall in venous pressure and arteriolar vasoconstriction was indicated by decreased blood flow of the hand. This study demonstrated how the nervous manifestations arise secondary to changes in the vascular system. The increase in heart rate, change in arterial pressure and vasoconstriction occurred instantly after tilting without subjective symptoms. The increase in pulse rate and the vasoconstrictor response were attributed to the stimulating effect of the lowered systolic pressure on the baroreceptor reflex mechanisms.

Table 4.1 Cardiac index, mean arterial pressure and peripheral resistance in 8 subjects before and during 60° head-up tilt faint. (Reprinted with permission from Arnold M. Weissler *et al.* and the American Heart Association, from *Circulation*, 1957, **15**: 875–882.)

Subject	Cardiac index (litres/min/m²)			Mean arterial pressure (mmHg)			Peripheral resistance (dyne-sec/cm⁵)		
	Control	Syncope	Change	Control	Syncope	Change	Control	Syncope	Change
GH	3.5	2.2	−1.3	100	38	−62	1128	689	−439
BW	2.5	1.6	−0.9	74	30	−44	1302	812	−490
BJ	3.2	2.5	−0.7	85	26	−59	1125	426	−699
DF	2.9	2.3	−0.6	80			1108		
LD	2.4	1.9	−0.5	82	55	−27	1407	1226	−181
JF	2.7	2.5	−0.2	87	57	−30	1358	956	−402
MS	2.2	2.5	+0.3	67	27	−40	1132	392	−740
LB	3.8	4.3	+0.5	95	32	−63	1064	320	−744
Mean	2.9	2.5	−0.4	84	38	−46	1217	689	−528
S.d.*			0.21						80
p			>0.05						<0.01

* Refers to standard error of the difference between means.
All data obtained while the subjects were in the 60° head-up tilt position.

The subsequent changes were attributed to increasing ischaemia of the medullary centres. Initially, hyperactivity of *both* sympathetic and parasympathetic functions occurred. With maximum medullary ischaemia the parasympathetic manifestations predominated. Initially, tachycardia, vasoconstriction, and dilated pupils were found simultaneously with sweating, yawning, belching, nausea, cramps (possibly pyloric spasm) and increased peristalsis. Immediately prior to the onset of syncope, bradycardia appeared. The sequence was tachycardia, fall in systolic pressure, reduced pulse pressure, arteriolar constriction, decreased blood flow in the hands, all preceding the symptoms of fainting. Circulatory collapse occurred when the maximum blood flow through the hands dropped to 20–40% of the normal value. Simultaneously, there was a fall in venous pressure usually reaching a level below that of the right atrium. (Weiss *et al.* used the second intercostal space and measured venous pressure by an indirect method. Their values should be increased by about 10 cmH_2O.) Further decrease in blood flow resulted in vasovagal syncope. Changes in the autonomic nervous system appeared as secondary manifestations to the primary action of nitrite on the peripheral vascular system. It is concluded that the simultaneous over-activity of the sympathetic and parasympathetic autonomic nervous systems arose first through peripheral vascular reflexes and was subsequently augmented by medullary ischaemia.

In another study of fainting induced by nitrites in normal subjects, Wilkins *et al.* (1937) found that fainting was accompanied by a fall in venous pressure and inadequate venous return.

Sodium nitrite is effective on the peripheral circulation in both prone and supine positions. It has been shown that the hands are distended by the same venous pressure from 20–40% more after nitrite than before. This decreased venous tone in the hand indicates that the venous side of the splanchnic circulation is not the sole site of blood pooling. In the upright position the arms and hands become blood depots as well as the feet, legs and abdominal viscera.

Sodium nitrite elicits a different pattern of vascular response in skeletal muscle than most dilator agents. There is a moderate dilatation of resistance vessels and a pronounced dilation of capacitance vessels in both cat and man. The pre- to post-capillary resistance ratio is unchanged by this drug and there is no significant net increase in transcapillary filtration because both pre- and post-capillary resistance vessels dilate. The relaxation of large arteries and especially the pronounced venous dilatation which can lead to an unloading of the heart, may help to explain the effects of nitrites in relieving angina.

Blood Pressure Changes and Respiration

A rise in blood pressure in the carotid sinus and aorta elicits a transient reflex decrease in rate and depth of breathing (Best and Taylor, 1980).

The opposite change is initiated by a sudden fall in pressure in these areas, i.e. hyperpnoea. Any sudden change in blood pressure tends to elicit a respiratory response, i.e. during rapid bleeding respiration is stimulated, an effect that is considerably reduced following sino-aortic denervation (Schopp *et al.*, 1957). Almost all slowly progressing vasovagal subjects who faint exhibit increased and deeper breathing before losing consciousness.

These changes in respiration can influence venous return (Youmans, 1958). The increased blood volume in the abdominal viscera during syncope is assisted out of the abdominal inferior cava into the thoracic portion by deeper breathing. Respiratory arrest during a rise in blood pressure favours pooling of blood in the splanchnic regions so that venous return is decreased as is cardiac output.

VASODILATATION IN MUSCLE

During emotional stress, blood pressure rises and blood is shifted from the splanchnic regions and skin to the muscles (Fencl *et al.*, 1959). Barcroft *et al.* (1960) have shown that stress induces vasodilatation of the vascular bed in muscle. Skin vessel changes were not constant and most often vasoconstriction. The vasodilatation was unrelated to arterial blood pressure which rose about 5% above resting levels during 4 min of mental arithmetic, while the mean forearm blood flow increased 225%.

Because the interval between the stimulus and the start of the vasodilatation may be either long or short, it has been suggested that both nervous and humoral agents are responsible for the forearm vasodilatation. As the vasodilatation persists after sympathectomy (although reduced) there must also be a humoral component.

The changes in forearm blood flow during 10 min of mental arithmetic or during a 10-min intravenous infusion of adrenaline were similar and as the vasodilatation was less after adrenalectomy, it was suggested that adrenaline might be involved.

Forearm blood flow after stellate ganglion block was less than before, suggesting a nervous mechanism. It was also less after intravenous atropine and after local brachial artery atropinization of the forearm relative to the control forearm. This is consistent with the theory of sympathetic cholinergic vasodilator fibres mediating emotionally-induced vasodilatation in muscle. This had also been shown by Blair *et al.* (1959).

Thus, muscular vasodilatation in the forearm during mental stress is mediated both by humoral substances and/or by sympathetic cholinergic fibres. This study concluded by noting the similarities between the haemodynamic reaction to mental stress in man and the reaction produced by stimulation of the hypothalamic zone in animals.

Passive Loss of Peripheral Resistance

A drop in blood pressure can occur due to *active* reflex loss of peripheral resistance and also due to *passive* loss. The passive loss is not the same as pooling. In the upright position, after a relatively short time, it is necessary to have contraction of leg muscles and an increase in their tone to aid venous return. Prolonged strapping to a tilt table will result in fainting in a certain number of subjects and prolonged immobilization in the upright position is probably the cause of death in crucifixion. In a group of healthy young people following vigorous exercise and then strapped to a tilt table, hypotension occurred in half and fainting in a quarter (Eichna *et al.*, 1947). Stead and Ebert (1941) pointed out that patients with postural hypotension do not pool more blood, but normal pooling causes an abnormal fall in blood pressure due to the *absence of vasoconstriction*.

Body Heating, Adrenaline and Forearm Blood Flow

Barcroft *et al.* (1947) also examined the effect of body heating on skeletal muscle blood flow. Body warming increased the blood flow in the forearm on the average from 3.1 to 9.3 ml per 100 ml forearm per minute. This change did not occur in sympathectomized forearms, confirming the earlier work of Wilkins and Eichna (1941) that it was a vascular reflex mediated by the sympathetic system. Furthermore, body warming increased the blood flow in the forearm when the skin blood vessels were constricted by adrenaline. It was concluded therefore that the dilatation was deep to the skin, probably in muscles.

In addition, Allen *et al.* (1946) observed the effects of adrenaline on human skeletal muscle blood flow. The adrenaline was infused intravenously and intra-arterially while the pulse rate, blood pressure and blood flow in the forearm, calf and hand were studied in normal and sympathectomized subjects. During the intravenous infusion, the blood flow in the forearm increased 4–5 fold in the first 2 min and then subsided to twice the resting rate during the third minute and thereafter remained constant until the end of the infusion. Qualitatively similar changes took place in the heart rate. The initial vasodilatation and that following constriction in the limb were unrelated to cardiac function. They were due to the action of the adrenaline in the limb as similar changes in the calf blood flow took place during infusion of adrenaline into the femoral artery, while heart rate and arterial blood pressure remained constant. The changes occurred in sympathectomized limbs, demonstrating that central vasomotor reflexes were not involved.

PLASMA VOLUME

Tarazi *et al.* (1970) examined plasma volume changes during 50° head-up tilt in 11 normal and 15 hypertensive subjects. No difference was found between the two groups. The capillary filtration rate in the first 5 min of tilt was greater than the rate over the entire 20 min of the tilt. There was no relationship between filtration rate and changes in mean arterial pressure, suggesting a dissociation between mechanisms regulating capillary exchange and those responsible for maintenance of systemic resistance. In the six patients who fainted during the tilt, the plasma volume changes were not different from those who did not.

ANTIDIURETIC HORMONE (ADH, VASOPRESSIN)

Davies and Forsling (1975) studied vasopressin release after postural change-induced syncope. They investigated plasma argipressin (arginine-vasopressin, AVP) in 12 volunteers tilted to 85° for 60 min. Blood pressure, pulse, and hematocrit, plasma AVP, renin and cortisol were monitored. Seven subjects completed the study, while five fainted. In the non-fainters, hematocrit rose from 32 to 47, plasma AVP rose from 1.1 to 5.2 and plasma cortisol did not change. In those who fainted, plasma cortisol rose significantly after the syncope. Plasma AVP showed a much more pronounced increase rising from 1.1 to 11 after fainting. The reported antidiuretic response accompanying syncope is at least in part due to an increased concentration of AVP in the circulation.

Davies *et al.* (1976) have also studied the responses of AVP and plasma renin to postural changes in normal subjects with particular attention to syncope. They used 14 mildly dehydrated, normal, subjects. They were slowly tilted at a constant rate from the horizontal to 85° head-up position.

Nine subjects did *not* develop vasovagal symptoms and were observed for 45–60 min. Argipressin rose in two phases in all subjects. A small initial rise was seen at 3 min and persisted for 30 min. This was followed by a striking rise between 30 min and 45 min when the fall of plasma volume had reached its maximum (17%). Plasma renin activity reached a maximum at 30 min, but fell by 45 min as plasma concentration of AVP rose.

Five subjects developed vasovagal symptoms, 4 to 24 min after reaching 85° when the study was terminated. There was a striking increase of AVP concentration within 4 min of syncope, but no change in plasma osmolality, cortisol concentration or renin activity occurred. Davies *et al.* suggested that the increase in plasma AVP was due to the isosmotic fall of plasma volume and may have been influenced by emotional factors as well. The trigger for the AVP release is uncertain. It may be intrathoracic volume receptors or related to brief periods of hypoxia. The same phenomenon is seen in mountain sickness. Acute hypoxia can lead to an antidiuresis in conscious subjects. Plasma cortisol concentration and renin activity do not increase. The increase of plasma AVP within 4 min of syncope is striking and seems related to the sensitive mechanisms for the preservation of the circulating volume.

Baylis and Heath (1977) have also measured plasma AVP concentrations in five healthy volunteers during postural changes under conditions of dehydration and normal hydration. A rise in plasma AVP was observed only after dehydration and standing for 40 min. Five further volunteers who developed pre-syncopal symptoms during orthostasis had extremely high plasma AVP levels. The changes in plasma AVP concentrations occurred with no alterations in plasma osmolality.

Baylis *et al.* (1978) have also studied the influence of lower-body negative pressure on AVP release. Lower-body negative pressure (9–12 kPa) was applied to 10 normal subjects. Large increases in plasma AVP concentration occurred only in those with syncopal symptoms and hypotension. Blood from the superior vena cava at half-minute intervals during application of the negative pressure showed that maximal plasma vasopressin concentrations occurred with hypotension.

HYPOXIA

Anderson *et al.* (1946) studied the mechanisms of hypoxic fainting in 13 normal subjects. They found increased forearm flow in hypoxic as well as in post-haemorrhagic fainting, indicating that active vasodilatation in skeletal muscle was a constant component of both types of syncope.

DECREASED BLOOD VOLUME AND POST-HAEMORRHAGIC SYNCOPE

Barcroft and Edholm (1945) induced fainting with tourniquets on the thighs and venesection. This caused fainting in 28 of 32 subjects. They then studied blood flow in the normal forearm and hand, in the sympathectomized and in the nerve-blocked forearm. During fainting, blood flow in the forearm increased as the arterial pressure fell, suggesting regional vasodilatation. Blood flow through the hand, which is mostly skin and bone, decreased indicating the forearm vasodilatation was in muscle. Sympathectomy abolished the forearm vasodilatation implying it was an active process brought about by the vasomotor centre and sympathetic nervous system and that there must be sympathetic vasodilator fibres in the forearm muscles. The vasomotor centre probably excites vasodilatation in the arterioles of all skeletal muscles which could explain the sudden fall in the arterial blood pressure in fainting.

Post-haemorrhagic Syncope

Vasovagal fainting with a drop in blood pressure and a slow pulse is well recognized after blood loss. The incidence of fainting increases as the haemorrhage increases in volume. Fainting occurred in 4% of donors bled 440 ml and rose to 8.5% of donors when the volume was increased to 540 ml (Poles and Boycott, 1942). Acute experimental blood loss has been used to study the nature of syncope.

Bleeding from normal male volunteers of 800 and 1000 ml resulted in 11 out of 28 fainting and of those bled 1000–1200 ml, 15 of 29 fainted (Wallace and Sharpey-Schafer, 1941).

Barcroft *et al.* (1944) carried out venous section or produced similar effects by placing tourniquets around the thighs at diastolic pressures for about 20 minutes and then bleeding a small quantity. The thigh tourniquet will produce a fall of right atrial pressure and cardiac output almost identical to that induced by venous section (McMichael and Sharpey-Schafer, 1944). About 700 ml of blood may be trapped in the legs in this manner.

Observations 2 h after a mid-day meal in the supine position were made of cardiac output, forearm blood flow and right atrial pressure. Seven normal subjects who fainted after blood loss of about 1000 ml were studied. During the bleeding, the heart rate increased and cardiac output and right atrial pressure fell. Blood pressure was maintained at almost pre-bleeding level. Constriction and total peripheral resistance, therefore, must have increased. A few minutes after the end of the bleeding the blood pressure fell suddenly, pulse slowed and the faint occurred. During the faint the pulse slowed further, cardiac output and right atrial pressure began to increase and were higher than at the end of the bleeding, implying a great decrease in total peripheral resistance (Barcroft *et al.*, 1944).

Forearm Blood Flow

Five of six subjects studied by Barcroft *et al.* had an increase in forearm blood flow during fainting, the increase occurring simultaneously with the fall in blood pressure. During recovery, as blood pressure rose, the flow decreased in parallel. When rapid re-transfusion occurred by deflation of the thigh cuffs, the rise of blood pressure and decrease of forearm blood flow occurred simultaneously.

Barcroft *et al.* demonstrated that venesection plus upright tilt caused an initial rise in total peripheral resistance and heart rate while the blood pressure, right atrial pressure and cardiac output fell. Shortly before the faint, cardiac output and right atrial pressure began to rise and did not fall during the unconscious period. Total peripheral resistance, heart rate and blood pressure fell precipitously however, while forearm muscle flow increased, evidently through vasodilatation. The failure of cardiac output to fall in the face of a marked bradycardia and decrease in peripheral resistance at the onset of a faint has been confirmed by Warren *et al.* (1945) and Weissler (1957). In addition, there was no significant change in the stroke volume, circulation time or venous pressure.

The associated symptoms of bradycardia, weakness, sweating, nausea and pallor, are due to intense autonomic nervous system stimulation as is the vasodilatation and fall in blood pressure. Many of these changes persist after the blood pressure has returned to normal. In other kinds of syncope these phenomena are not present. The splanchnic and renal vascular beds also take part in the vasodilatation coinciding with the loss of consciousness (Bearn *et al.*, 1951; DeWardner and McSweeney, 1951).

Barcroft and Edholm (1945) thought that the diminished peripheral resistance due to peripheral vasodilatation was the cause of the acute fall in blood pressure. The vasodilatation demonstrated in the forearm blood flow was significant. Skin vessels were excluded as skin pallor was consistent with decreased blood flow.

Studies of blood flow in the forearm and calf of the leg (Grant and Pearson, 1938; Wilkins and Eichna, 1941) have shown that a given procedure affects both flows in the same direction. It seems possible that the vessels of all the skeletal musculature react in the same way, possibly varying only in degree.

The increased blood flow to muscles during faint is not the result of diminished resistance related to loss of muscle tone during the faint. Barcroft and Edholm (1945) blocked the motor nerve to the forearm muscles in two sympathectomized subjects and found that the paralysis did not increase forearm flow.

The following are reasonable suppositions on the mechanism of this type of syncope. The acute fall in blood pressure cannot be explained by heart slowing and decreased cardiac output. It is due to peripheral vasodilatation in muscle, and has been demonstrated in forearm muscle. If the same degree of vasodilatation occurred throughout the body musculature there would be a substantial drop in the blood pressure. The vasodilatation is mediated by vasomotor nerves. This vasodilatation in muscle is augmented by adrenaline (Grant and Pearson, 1938) which is known to rise during haemorrhage and is further increased by the diminished levels of arterial pCO_2 which apparently occurs in all faints of gradual onset.

Table 4.2 Synopsis of experimental syncope

- Experimental syncope induced by nitrites and head-up tilt is characterized by pre-syncopal symptoms before there is hypotension or bradycardia
- In this type of syncope there is a widespread loss of peripheral resistance, an insignificant drop in cardiac output, an unimportant bradycardia, and because of an unchanging venous return, a failure of cardiac output to compensate for the diminished peripheral resistance
- The tachypnoea which is a common pre-syncopal symptom is not of prime importance but does add to the peripheral vasodilatation of muscle and contributes to reducing cerebral blood flow
- Stress dilates the vascular bed in muscles by nervous and humoral mechanisms
- Syncope after haemorrhage, or haemorrhage and thigh tourniquets, is also due to decreased peripheral resistance from vasodilatation in muscle
- The pre-syncopal symptoms of pallor, nausea, weakness, sweating and epigastric distress occur before the hypotension and persist after the blood pressure returns to normal

Venesection and Thigh Tourniquet

Warren *et al.* (1945) have also used venesection and thigh tourniquets to provoke syncope in normal volunteers. The subjects (all normal) were studied by removing 309 ml of blood and/or placing thigh tourniquets. From their data it was evident that venous pressure at the level of the right atrium is in excess of that required in standing man, to adequately fill the heart.

Doupe *et al.* (1938) demonstrated the same thing. They emphasized that cardiac output may remain normal with a falling right atrial pressure and conversely, from a study of normal subjects, that anxiety can cause a striking rise in cardiac output without a rise in atrial pressure. In the three patients who fainted in this study there was a marked fall in systolic, diastolic and mean arterial pressure without change in cardiac output.

Clinical observation shows that pallor, epigastric distress, sweating, weakness and slow pulse may or may not be accompanied by a fall in blood pressure. In addition, these symptoms may persist long after the pressure has returned to normal. The sudden faint, heart block, or cardiac standstill from carotid sinus compression is not associated with these symptoms and patients with true orthostatic hypotension have a striking fall in blood pressure when upright. These patients do not have these symptoms as the blood pressure falls. All of these observations support the assumption that the entire syndrome of pallor, nausea, weakness, sweating, slow pulse, etc. and fall in blood pressure result from reflex stimulation of the autonomic nervous system and that the fall in arterial pressure accompanies rather than causes the other symptoms. The three normal subjects who had acute circulatory collapse plus the above symptoms had strikingly slow pulse, a marked fall in blood pressure and peripheral resistance. The right atrial pressure increased and the cardiac output remained unchanged. The circulatory collapse appeared to be the result of a sudden decrease in peripheral resistance due to reflex vasodilatation. There was no evidence of decreased venous return.

The salient features of experimental syncope are summarized in Table 4.2

REFERENCES

Allen WJ, Barcroft H and Edholm OG (1946) On the action of adrenaline on the blood vessels in human skeletal muscles. *Journal of Physiology* **105**: 255–267.

Anderson DP, Allen WJ, Barcroft H, Edholm OG and Manning GW (1946) Circulatory changes during fainting and coma caused by oxygen lack. *Journal of Physiology* **104**: 426–434.

Barcroft H, Bonner WM and Edholm OG (1947) Reflex vasodilatation in human skeletal muscle in response to heating the body. *Journal of Physiology* **106**: 271–278.

Barcroft H, Brod J, Hejl Z, Hirsjarvi EA and Kitchin AH (1960) The mechanism of the vasodilatation in the forearm muscles during stress. *Clinical Science* **19**: 577–586.

Barcroft H, Edholm OG, McMichael J and Sharpey-Schafer EP (1944) Posthaemorrhagic fainting. *Lancet* **1**: 489–491.

Barcroft H and Edholm OG (1945) On the vasodilatation in human skeletal muscle during post-haemorrhagic fainting. *Journal of Physiology* **104**: 161–175.

Baylis PH and Heath DA (1977) Influence of presyncope and postural change upon plasma arginine vasopressin concentration in hydrated and dehydrated man. *Clinical Endocrinology* **7**: 79–83.

Baylis PH, Stockley RA and Heath DA (1978) Influence of lower body negative pressure on arginine vasopressor release. *Clinical Endocrinology* **9**(1): 89–95.

Bearn AG, Billing D, Edholm OG and Sherlock S (1951) Hepatic blood flow and carbohydrate changes in man during fainting. *Journal of Physiology* **115**: 442–455.

Best CH and Taylor NB (1980) *Physiological Basis of Medical Practice*, 10th Edition, pp. 6–62. Baltimore: Williams and Wilkins.

Blair DA, Glover WE, Greenfield ADM and Roddie IC (1959) Excitation of cholinergic vasodilator nerves to human skeletal muscle during emotional stress. *Journal of Physiology* **148**: 633.

Davies R and Forsling ML (1975) Vasopressin release after postural changes and syncope. *Journal of Endocrinology* **65**(3): 59P–60P.

Davies R, Slater JDH, Forsling ML and Payne N (1976) The response of arginine vasopressin and plasma renin to postural changes in normal man with observations on syncope. *Clinical Science and Molecular Medicine* **51**: 267–274.

DeWardener HE and McSweeney RR (1951) Renal hemodynamics in vasovagal fainting due to hemorrhage. *Clinical Science* **10**: 209–217.

Doupe J, Krynauw RA and Snodgrass SR (1938) Some factors influencing venous pressure in man. *Journal of Physiology* **92**: 383–400.

Eichna LW, Horvath SM and Bean WB (1947) Post-exertional orthostatic hypotension. *American Journal of Medicine* **213**: 641.

Fencl V, Hejl Z, Jirka J, Madlafousek J and Brod J (1959) Changes in blood flow in forearm muscle and skin during acute emotional stress (mental arithmetic). *Clinical Science* **18**: 491.

Gilman AG, Goodman LS and Gilman A (1980) *The Pharmacologic Basis of Therapeutics*, 6th Edition, pp. 820–822. New York: MacMillan.

Grant RT and Pearson RSB (1938) The blood circulation in the human limb. Observations on the differences between the proximal and distal parts and remarks on the regulation of body temperature. *Clinical Science* **3**: 119–139.

McMichael J and Sharpey-Schafer EP (1944) Cardiac output in man by a direct Fick method. *British Heart Journal* **6**: 33.

Poles FC and Boycott M (1942) Syncope in blood donors. *Lancet* **2**: 531–535.

Schopp RT, Gilfoil TM and Youmans WB (1957) Mechanisms of respiratory responses to vasodilator drugs, urecholine and nitroglycerin. *American Journal of Physiology* **189**: 123–128.

Stead EA and Ebert RV (1941) Postural hypotension, a disease of the sympathetic nervous system. *Archives of Internal Medicine* **67**: 546.

Tarazi RC, Melsher HJ, Dustan HP and Frohlich ED (1970) Plasma volume changes with upright tilt: studies in hypertension and in syncope. *Journal of Applied Physiology* **28**(2): 121–126.

Wallace J and Sharpey-Schafer EP (1941) Blood changes following controlled haemorrhage in man. *Lancet* **2**: 393–395.

Warren JV, Brannon ES, Stead EA and Merrill AJ (1945) The effect of venesection and the pooling of blood in the extremities on the atrial pressure and cardiac output in normal subjects with observations on acute circulatory collapse in three instances. *Journal of Clinical Investigation* **24**: 337–344.

Weiss S, Wilkins RW and Haynes FW (1937) The nature of circulatory collapse induced by sodium nitrite. *Journal of Clinical Investigation* **16**: 73–84.

Weissler AM, Warren JV, Estes EH, McIntosh HD and Leonard JJ (1957) Vasodepressor syncope—factors influencing cardiac output. *Circulation* **15**: 875–882.

Wilkins RW and Eichna LW (1941) Blood flow to forearm and calf. Vasomotor reactions: role of sympathetic nervous system. *Johns Hopkins Hospital Bulletin* **68**: 450.

Wilkins RW, Haynes FW and Weiss S (1937) The role of the venous system in circulatory collapse induced by sodium nitrite. *Journal of Clinical Investigation* **16**: 85–91.

Williams JK, Glick G and Braunwald E (1965) Studies on cardiac dimensions in intact unanaesthetized man. Effects of nitroglycerin. *Circulation* **32**: 767–771.

Youmans WB (1958) Role of respiratory response to changes in arterial blood pressure. *Anaesthesiology* **19**: 552–554 (editorial).

5

Cardiac Syncope

INTRODUCTION

Syncope without warning is almost always cardiac in origin, although many cases of cardiac syncope are of gradual onset.

Atrio-ventricular heart block or cardiac dysrhythmia are the commonest causes of cardiac syncope. The heart block may be fixed or intermittent and preceded by right, left, or bilateral bundle branch block. Fainting occurs when the block becomes complete and an idioventricular pacemaker **below** the block fails to function for more than a few seconds (Friedberg, 1971). The subsequent ventricular rhythm may be standstill or a burst of ventricular fibrillation (rare). It may subside on its own in 10 or 15 sec with a return of idioventricular pacemaker or sinus rhythm.

Less common syncope related to cardiac standstill may be due to sinus arrest or sino-atrial block. The syncope can appear without warning in a patient with regular sinus rhythm and a normal ECG or with sinus bradycardia between attacks. The attacks may occur unrelated to any disease and may be due to various drugs such as quinidine (Friedberg, 1971).

Syncope may also be due to cardiac standstill at the onset of paroxysmal supraventricular arrhythmias. This may be symptomatic of functional deficiency of the sinus node or sino-atrial conduction and a component of the bradycardia–tachycardia syndrome.

Cardiac syncope is an indication for a demand or fixed-rate pacemaker. The electrode is usually placed in the right ventricle, although a right atrial pacemaker may be preferable if there is no disturbance in atrioventricular conduction. If syncope is proven to follow atrial fibrillation or other supraventricular tachycardia, digitalis may prevent it. If due to recurrent ventricular tachycardia and/or fibrillation, procainamide or quinidine alone or in combination with propranolol may be given prophylactically. If drugs are ineffective, a pacemaker must be inserted although drugs may still be necessary and may be given with greater safety after insertion of a pacemaker.

Syncope and/or sudden death may occur in patients with cardiomyopathies, with conduction disturbances, and in families, particularly in young people with documented ventricular fibrillation during the attack and with congenital defects of the conduction system shown at autopsy. *The syncope may follow severe exertion or acute mental stress.*

Syncope with ventricular fibrillation and sudden death are part of the childhood syndrome of Jervell and Lange–Nielsen (surdocardiac syndrome). This is characterized by congenital

Table 5.1 Major ECG abnormalities in 122 043 asymptomatic US Air Force personnel. (From Hiss and Lamb (1962) and reproduced by permission from A. J. Dunning (1979) *Cerebral Manifestations of Episodic Cardiac Dysrhythmias* (ed. E. W. Busse). Princeton: Excerpta Medica.

	Rate per 1000
Atrial rhythm	5.5
Atrial premature beats	4.3
Nodal premature beats	2.1
Ventricular premature beats	7.8
First-degree AV block	6.5
W–P–W syndrome	1.5
Right bundle branch block	1.8
AV dissociation	0.7

deafness and a prolonged QT interval. Syncope may also occur in the incomplete syndrome in which there is a long QT interval and no deafness (see Chapter 8).

Abnormal Heart Rhythm and Asymptomatic People

In the investigation of syncope abnormalities of cardiac function will be found frequently. These same abnormalities are also commonly present in the asymptomatic public. The task in the diagnosis of cardiac syncope is to document the abnormality of heart rate or rhythm at the time of a syncopal attack.

The definition of normal heart function is not as clear as one might expect. The electrocardiograms of 122 000 apparently healthy males (US Air Force) from 16 to 50 years of age were abnormal in about 5%. The commonest rhythm abnormalities found are shown in Table 5.1 (Hiss and Lamb, 1962).

Another study assessed 301 healthy, middle-aged men, with 6 h of taped ECG recording during ordinary daily activities (Hinkle *et al.*, 1969). Six percent had defects of conduction either fixed or intermittent. There was a high incidence of supraventricular and ventricular premature beats and dysrhythmias (62%) (Table 5.2). Although only 39 of 301 subjects had overt coronary artery disease, the ventricular arrhythmias or premature contractions or conduction defects were significantly related to the risk of subsequent death from coronary heart disease.

Sleep

The neurophysiological trigger of *awakening* seems to be an important factor in the apparent random provocation of premature ventricular beats, rather than a reflection of the state of the heart itself (Dunning, 1979). There is a marked divergence of opinion on the effect of *sleep* on cardiac rhythm.

Lown *et al.* (1973) recorded cardiac rhythm in 54 subjects, 31 with stable coronary artery disease and 12 who were normal. A 50% reduction in the number and complexity of ventricular premature beats was seen during sleep in both groups on repeated occasions. It was more marked in the normal subjects who usually lost all ectopic ventricular activity. Drug

Table 5.2 Rhythm and conduction abnormalities without symptoms in 301 active middle-aged males during a 6-h recording period. (Hinkle *et al.* (1969) and reproduced with permission from A. J. Dunning (1979) *Cerebral Manifestations of Episodic Cardiac Dysrhythmias* (ed. E. W. Busse). Princeton: Excerpta Medica.

Recordings with	Supraventricular		Ventricular
1 or more premature beats	76.0%		62.2%
Less than 1 per 1000 complexes	63.2%		33.9%
1–10 per 1000 complexes	6.4%		19.4%
> 10 per 1000 complexes	6.4%		8.8%
Paroxysmal tachycardia	0.7%		3.2%
Complex dysrhythmias (paired, multiple, bigeminy)	17.7%		19.1%
Sinoatrial block		1.4%	
Atrioventricular block		0.7%	
Intraventricular block		7.7%	

treatment was inferior to sleep in suppressing ventricular activity in a number of patients. In contrast, Lopez *et al.* (1975) found a 13% occurrence of new ventricular arrhythmias during sleep. The abnormalities recorded during the day decreased markedly during sleep in more than 60% of their patients with coronary heart disease. In both groups, however, supraventricular arrhythmias increased during sleep.

Clarke *et al.* (1976) monitored the heart rate and rhythm of 101 apparently normal office workers. Each had a complete medical examination and two 24-h ECG recordings. All subjects with any abnormalities or on any medication except oral contraceptives were excluded.

The heart rate over the entire 24-h period was significantly higher in females, ranging from 85 to 95 beats during the day down to 65 during sleep (Fig. 5.1). The heart rate in males was five beats slower with no relationship between heart rate and age and the rate was significantly higher in smokers than non-smokers in both sexes.

Seven subjects had more than five ventricular ectopic beats per hour (over the 48 h) and four were multifocal. Two subjects with ventricular tachycardia were observed, all without symptoms and unrelated to any recorded event. In 10 other subjects, brady-arrhythmias were seen, two with second degree atrioventricular block during sleep and eight with episodes of nodal rhythm while awake or asleep. All the recorded events were asymptomatic. A repeat Holter monitoring of the group about 15 months after the initial study revealed a similar level of abnormality (Shelton, 1986).

From these studies it appears that some arrhythmias, particularly of ventricular origin, indicate a bad prognosis (i.e. sudden death) in patients with heart disease. Their importance is unknown in apparently healthy people but it appears to be minimal.

Age and physical condition are important contributors to bradycardia. In 50 healthy medical students the minimal heart rate during sleep was 33–55/min. Sinus arrhythmia with doubling of the preceding cycle length was seen in half of the subjects. Sinus pauses of nearly 2 sec were seen and frequent atrial and ventricular premature beats were common (Brodsky *et al.*, 1977).

The variations of rhythm of the normal healthy heart are large and overlap the common dysrhythmias of the diseased or aging heart. It is often difficult to determine the significance of arrhythmias and conduction disturbances found in healthy and sick people.

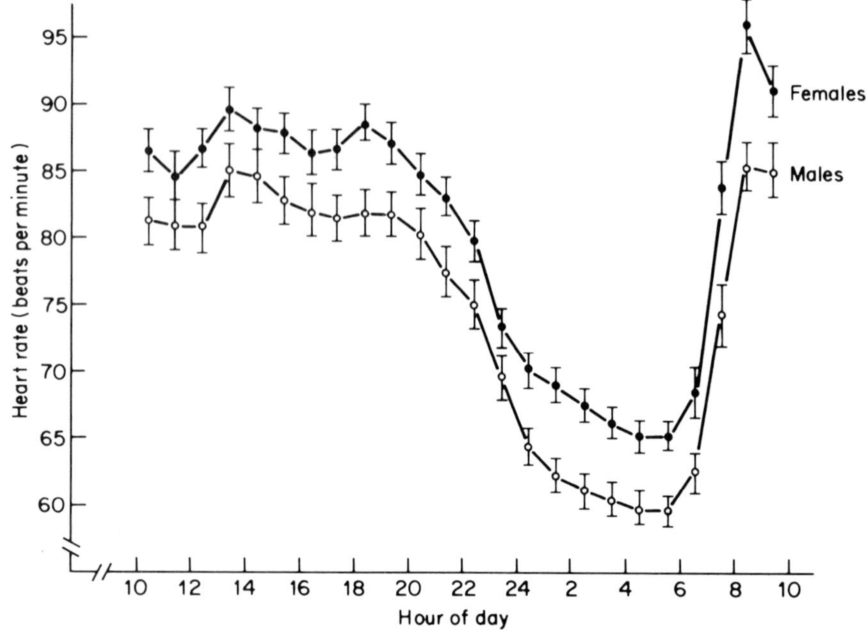

Figure 5.1 Average circadian rhythm of heart rate, male and female (mean ± S.E.M.). (Reproduced with permission from J. M. Clarke and *Lancet*, 1976, **2**: 509.)

Finally, there is some individual variation in the tolerance of arrhythmia and asystole. Stern and Tzivoni (1976) reported a patient with asystole for 19–20 sec. This produced dizziness but not unconsciousness.

INTERMITTENT DISTURBANCES OF RHYTHM

The episodic arrhythmias which may be related to cerebral symptoms are:

1. Sino-atrial bradycardia—the sick sinus syndrome ('brady–tachy' syndrome)
2. Atrioventricular block
3. Complex ventricular arrhythmias

Bradycardia

Bradycardia and tachycardia can be two aspects of the same disease and part of the 'brady–tachy' syndrome. Bradycardia of less than 30/min is usually better tolerated than tachycardia of more than 150/min. A slow heart has a longer filling time and a greater stroke volume. As cardiac output is a combination of stroke volume and rate, and increase of the former can compensate for a bradycardia.

Bradycardia is not necessarily pathological at any age. Twenty-four hour ambulatory ECG recordings in 20 young, male, long-distance runners during activity other than running revealed an average waking heart rate of 46 ± 6/min. Heart rates in the low 30s were the norm during sleep. Asymptomatic sinus pauses up to 2.7 sec were present. In 40% of the subjects, some degree of atrioventricular block with Wenckebach periods was found (Talan *et al.*, 1982). Hanson and Tabakin (1965) have also found the resting rate in athletes to be as slow as 36–40/min. Bradycardia in athletes is generally thought to be due to increased vagal tone and decreased sympathetic activity and blunted sympathetic responsiveness. Profound asymptomatic bradycardia in well-conditioned athletes may be normal (see Chapter 13).

Sino-atrial Bradycardia

Sino-atrial bradycardia may result from digitalis, quinidine or propranolol, and diseases such as myxoedema. Hyperkalaemia or hypokalaemia may produce bradycardia. Vagal stimulation secondary to increased intracranial pressure, oesophageal diverticulum, or carotid sinus compression is another mechanism.

Fowler *et al.* (1970) described six patients, age 50–74 years, with chronic symptomatic sino-atrial bradycardia. None had more than first degree atrioventricular block. The cause of the bradycardia was unknown except in one who had coronary artery disease and a myocardial infarction. Five of the six suffered from syncope. In three the syncope was due to cardiac slowing or arrest. Cardiac pacing was effective in all. Chronic sino-atrial bradycardia is much less common than atrioventricular block as a cause of cardiogenic syncope but must be considered in the differential diagnosis of fainting.

Sinus bradycardia has been accepted as a physiological finding in the aged. Of 98 elderly patients evaluated by monitoring, 11 had resting heart rates below 50/min. Ectopic rhythms and tachycardia were also relatively common in this apparently healthy group (Camm *et al.*, 1980).

Differentiating between the extremes of physiological sinus bradycardia and sinus node dysfunction is not simple.

Sino-atrial Syncope, 'Brady–Tachy' Syndrome, the Sick Sinus Syndrome

In 1954 Short described four patients with *alternating* bradycardia and supraventricular tachycardia associated with syncope. They had sinus rates of 22 to 48 beats/min with periods of 'sinus standstill' in two of them.

Birchfield *et al.* (1957) and Von Herbinger (1961) described similar patients with bradycardia, asystole, paroxysmal atrial fibrillation and syncope.

From these reports and others (Adelman and Wigle, 1969) a well-defined syndrome, sino-atrial syncope, has emerged. It consists of syncope due to sino-atrial block and bradycardia in addition to a variety of supraventricular tachycardias, usually paroxysmal atrial fibrillation or flutter.

The abnormality in sino-atrial syncope is not only the bradycardia, refractory to exercise and drugs, plus the supraventricular tachycardia; it is also the failure of the normal atrial and atrioventricular junctional escape pacemaker to take over. The latter fires at less than 60 beats/min and usually becomes the effective pacer when sino-atrial pacemakers fail. If this does not happen, more primitive idioventricular pacemakers will maintain cardiac rhythm or else asystole occurs.

The sino-atrial node is the primary pacemaker of the heart. It may be abnormal in impulse formation or conduction. It may be involved in a disease process but is more commonly abnormal due to degenerative lesions of unknown aetiology (Ferrer, 1973).

Acute or chronic coronary artery disease may produce sinus node dysfunction. Shillington and Thomas (1968) report that up to 20% of patients with acute myocardial infarctions may have sinus bradycardia. Other causes are cardiomyopathy, neuromuscular disorders, sarcoid, collagen disease and amyloid. In this syndrome atrial bradycardia or asystole alternating with paroxysmal tachycardia is common and the combination is referred to as the bradycardia–tachycardia ('brady–tachy') syndrome. A common presentation is via rate-related cerebral symptoms. The essence of the syndrome is an abnormal sino-atrial node with impaired pacemaker activity.

The sick sinus syndrome is both chronic and intermittent. It features sinus bradycardia, periods of sinus arrest, or sino-atrial block and tachycardia (Lown, 1967). The arrhythmias may occur in any sequence and dizziness and syncope are common symptoms (Rubenstein *et al.*, 1972). Transient neurological symptoms are less common (Abdon and Malcrona, 1975) as are systemic emboli (Rubenstein *et al.*, 1972).

Sutton and Perrins (1979) described 37 patients with the sick sinus syndrome. Their ECG abnormalities were intermittent sinus bradycardia, sino-atrial block or sinus arrest (spontaneous or during carotid sinus massage) with supraventricular tachycardia or atrial fibrillation. Electrophysiological studies revealed prolonged sinus node recovery after atrial pacing (Narula *et al.*, 1972). The mean age of the patients at diagnosis was 68 years with a range of 36–89 years and the female to male ratio was 1.4:1.

Symptoms (from Sutton and Perrins, 1979)

Brief syncope. The presenting symptoms were Adams–Stokes attacks, syncope or near syncope, in 22 patients with an average duration of 2.9 years. The unconscious episodes usually came without warning and often resulted in injury. They were occasionally preceded by pain, palpitation, or dyspnoea but these symptoms generally occurred after regaining consciousness. There was great variation in the frequency and duration of attacks. Only two patients had further syncopal episodes after the installation of a pacemaker. In one, the syncope was related to exit block and in the other to a tachycardia which responded to propranolol. Both had ventricular pacers. Four other patients had dizzy spells after pacing but of reduced frequency. These were related to episodic tachycardia and required anti-arrhythmic drugs.

Syncope occurs in 25–70% of patients with sinus node dysfunction (Medina and Dreifus, 1983). In 828 patients syncope was present in 59% presenting with the 'brady–tachy' syndrome, in 45% of patients presenting with sinus arrest and/or sino-atrial block and in 33% of patients presenting with persistent sinus bradycardia only. Two-thirds of the patients had organic heart disease including 56% with ischaemic heart disease. Syncope occurred in 48% of the 828 patients and was the commonest cause for hospitalization (Simonsen *et al.*, 1980).

Easley and Goldstein (1971) described 13 patients with cardiac syncope due to disordered sino-atrial conduction and depression of the atrioventricular junctional escape pacemaker. Significant atrioventricular block was not present in these patients. Two mechanisms of cardiac slowing were identified. Type I sino-atrial syncope was present in six patients with severe sino-atrial block and bradycardia. Type II sino-atrial syncope was present in seven patients. They had episodes of bradycardia/tachycardia, with asystole and syncope occurring at the end of the tachycardia. In one patient, the episodes were transient after an acute myocardial infarction. In 12 patients, the sino-atrial syncope was a chronic recurrent problem and in 11 of these it was successfully treated with ventricular demand pacing.

Neurological symptoms were present in 12 patients and had a mean duration of four years.

Extended syncope. Three patients had premonitory symptoms and were unconscious for up to $1\frac{1}{2}$ h. Bradycardia was the precipitating arrhythmia in all. A classical example was the description of a 71-year-old male with three attacks in 16 months (Sutton and Perrins, 1979): 'When I have an attack there is a feeling of coldness all over my body. This is followed by sweating and I lie down. I am then unconscious for 40 to 45 minutes and am exhausted for several hours afterwards. My wife says I am grey during the attack. I have also had brief dizzy spells for the previous five years following an inferior myocardial infarction. There have been no attacks since ventricular pacing'.

Epileptic seizures. These occurred in two patients. One had attacks without warning and had been unconscious for 40 min at a time. The other patient had syncope without warning followed by a generalized convulsion and amnesia lasting 2 h. The attacks were abolished by pacing.

Focal neurological symptoms. These were the only symptoms in one patient. A transient hemiparesis occurred in one patient, hemiparesis after syncope in another patient, dizziness and visual disturbance in two, and dizziness, syncope, with transient paraesthesiae or monoparesis in three additional patients. Typical histories were as follows:

> Mrs F. S., aged 71 years, four attacks in 18 months. 'At the start I feel tired. My speech is abnormal, I sound as though I am drunk. The left side of my face becomes weak. I am unsteady on my feet and feel lopsided. After the attack my face flushes.' Syncope did not occur and bradycardia was documented by her son, a doctor.
>
> Mr H. T., aged 64 years, attacks every week for two years. 'I start to sweat, my eyesight is affected. It is like looking down a tunnel. I am dizzy, I have to lie down. I become unconscious for five or 10 minutes and I feel exhausted for two to three hours afterwards. I am troubled by palpitations.' These symptoms and asystole were reproduced by left carotid massage producing asystole and abolished by pacing.

Chest pain, palpitations, and dyspnoea. These were the presenting features in only two patients. In both cases the pain was associated with intense sinus bradycardia. Chest pain was also frequently present as an associated symptom in 23 other patients. Palpitation was the presenting symptom in only one patient. It was occasionally associated with diplopia and was due to supraventricular tachycardia. Dyspnoea was a commonly associated symptom.

Diagnosis

ECG. The resting ECG was consistently normal in only three patients. Sinus bradycardia was the most common abnormality and was present in 26. Sino-atrial block was seen in 21, tachycardia, or atrial fibrillation in 14. Ischaemic changes were evident in 14 and five of these had a previous infarct. No anterior infarctions were seen. Fascicular or first degree atrioventricular block was present in 10, and only two had prolonged HV times revealed at His bundle electrography. Sinus node recovery was abnormal in 18 of 21. There was a higher incidence of associated conduction disturbances in other series (Ferrer, 1968; Rubenstein *et al.*, 1972).

Graded exercise. This was performed in 19 patients; 13 of these failed to achieve a heart rate above 120 beats per minute at maximum exercise. This was a higher positive yield in relation to identification of the sick sinus syndrome than that obtained by 24-h ECG recordings where only 10 of 16 patients were positive. Repeated resting ECGs, graded exercise testing, and 24-h Holter monitoring, will usually make the diagnosis. If not, electrophysiological studies to determine the sinus node recovery time are required. Permanent pacing was a safe, effective, treatment of symptomatic sick sinus syndrome irrespective of the presenting symptom (Sutton and Perrins, 1979).

Atrioventricular Block and Bundle Branch Block

Some kinds of atrioventricular (AV) block are present in the asymptomatic population and are relatively common in any group of well-trained athletes. They may be considered unimportant. The varieties of AV block are:

First degree—a simple delay in AV conduction as manifest by a P–R interval longer than 0.20 sec. It may be in the AV node, the His bundle, or the bundle branches.

Second degree—an episodic interruption in the conduction through the AV conducting tissues. It may be regular or irregular and may have progressively increasing P–R intervals (Mobitz Type I), fixed (Mobitz Type II), or variable P–R intervals.

Third degree—is a total interruption of conduction between atria and ventricles.

First-degree AV block was found in 11 of 126 healthy athletes (Meytes *et al.*, 1975).

The Mobitz Type I second-degree block is usually in the AV node, is preceded by an increasing P–R interval (The Wenckebach Periodicity phenomenon), and is of good prognosis. It can be drug-induced and was present in three of the athletes described by Meytes *et al.* (1975).

Mobitz Type II second-degree block is never normal, is more commonly in the His–Purkinje system as reflected by a wide QRS complex in the ECG, and has a high correlation with syncopal symptoms. There is also a high incidence of third-degree block in these patients (Dreifus and Watanabe, 1971) and a high correlation with sudden severe vertigo and/or unconsciousness.

Below the AV node the intraventricular conducting system has three distinct fascicles.

1. The right-bundle branch
2. The left-bundle branch—an anterior fascicle
3. The left-bundle branch—a posterior fascicle.

A bifascicular block may be right-bundle branch block with left-anterior hemi-block or complete left-bundle branch block. Trifascicular block is the addition of a prolonged AV conduction time.

Often chronic AV block is not a manifestation of coronary or other types of heart disease

(Dunning, 1979). In this author's series of 250 patients with chronic AV block the mean age at pacemaker implantation was 74 years, well above the average life expectancy of the community. Apparently degeneration or fibrosis of the distal conduction system may be an isolated cardiac abnormality and a pacemaker can keep these patients alive and symptom-free for years.

Symptoms of chronic AV block are intermittent and may be infrequent. Major conduction disturbances without symptoms are extremely common in the aged population (Dreifus and Watanabe, 1971).

Dunning *et al.* (1979) found first- and second-degree AV block, right- and left-bundle branch block, and left-anterior hemi-block in 51 of 100 healthy subjects.

Syncope in patients with bifascicular or trifascicular block suggests progression of the conduction defect to third-degree complete AV block and this progression has been documented in some cases.

Five hundred and fifty-four patients with chronic bifascicular and trifascicular conduction block were followed for three years (McAnulty *et al.*, 1982). Of the 160 deaths, 42 were sudden and most of these were due to tachyarrhythmias and myocardial infarctions. The major predictor of sudden death was the underlying heart disease, not the bundle branch block. However, a prolonged P–R interval indicated an increased risk of sudden death.

Bifascicular or trifascicular block in patients with a history of syncope is not necessarily an ominous finding (Medina and Dreifus, 1983).

In 186 patients with this diagnosis, the 30 patients with syncope did well. Only six had bradyarrhythmias preventable by pacing. In the other 24 patients, either no cause for syncope was found or they were not helped by pacing. The risk of sudden death in patients with syncope was the same as in other patients with similar bundle branch block but without syncope (Dhingra *et al.*, 1974).

Tachycardia

Tachycardia is a less common cause of severe vertigo and syncope than sino-atrial or AV block, or bradycardia.

Tachycardia may be sinus, atrial nodal or ventricular in origin and the commoner nonspecific symptoms are breathlessness, retrosternal discomfort and apprehension at onset. Some patients with tachycardia will faint because of the tachycardia, only if they suddenly assume the upright position. Tachycardia may occur when there is no other evidence of heart disease or as a manifestation of severe heart disease.

The diagnosis of tachycardia causing pre-syncopal symptoms or syncope is dependent on the dysrhythmia occurring while the patient is being examined or monitored.

Silent arrhythmias including tachycardia are common in the normal population as exemplified by the study of Zeldis *et al.* (1980). They assessed 477 patients with 24-h ECG recordings. The patients had assorted cardiovascular complaints but the correlation between symptoms and rhythm disturbances was only 13%. In addition, they found that 44 of 54 recorded episodes of supraventricular tachycardia and 37 of 40 episodes of ventricular tachycardia were symptom-free.

Postural Heart Block

Not all patients who become vertiginous and syncopal when changing from the supine to

Table 5.3 Obstructive heart diseases

Left heart
Aortic stenosis—congenital or acquired
Idiopathic hypertrophic subaortic stenosis (IHSS)
Prothetic valve malfunction*
Myxoma
Right heart
Eisenmenger syndrome
Tetralogy of Fallot
Primary pulmonary hypertension (see Chapter 9)
Pulmonary emboli (see Chapter 9)
Pulmonary stenosis

* Not discussed in this chapter.

upright have idiopathic orthostatic hypotension or autonomic failure. Seda *et al.* (1980) described a 53-year-old man with dizziness and syncope on standing. This was due to intermittent, Type II second-degree AV block, which occurred only when he was upright. It could not be precipitated by carotid sinus massage or prevented by the administration of atropine.

Left atrial myxoma causes syncope by obstructing cardiac output and this syncope can also occur with changes in posture.

Obstructive Heart Disease

Patients with any of the diseases in Table 5.3 may have syncope at rest or more commonly on effort. The mechanisms of the syncope are many and mentioned with the more common types of obstructive heart disease.

Aortic stenosis

Syncope with effort is an important symptom in this disease as it may be with any valvular heart disease. There are several factors contributing to the syncopal attacks.

The thought, as well as the start, of effort or exercise will dilate the vascular bed in muscle (see Chapter 13). This *decrease* in peripheral resistance plus the failure of cardiac output to increase are part of the mechanisms of syncope. Transient arrhythmias, relative myocardial ischaemia and failure, as well as a further drop in peripheral resistance mediated from cardiac baroreceptors will also contribute to reduced cerebral blood flow and syncope (Schwartz *et al.*, 1969; Mark *et al.*, 1973).

The syncope of aortic stenosis with exercise occurs at any age, and may be associated with angina and sudden death (Schwartz *et al.*, 1969). Ross and Braunwald (1968) found the average survival in aortic stenosis was three years following the onset of syncope. In the nine adult patients with this disease studied by Schwartz *et al.* (1969) the syncopal loss of consciousness was associated with a sudden drop in blood pressure, pallor, absent pulses and the disappearance of the aortic murmur.

If the syncopal spells were less than 40 sec, the ECG revealed a sinus rhythm with changes in the QRS complexes and ST segments. If longer than 40 sec, the ECG revealed whole heart or ventricular standstill or ventricular flutter or fibrillation. In addition, ECG evidence of diminished coronary blood flow was evident.

Idiopathic Hypertrophic Subaortic Stenosis

This condition may be part of Friedreich's ataxia, myotonic dystrophy or can occur independently. Syncope occurs in about 30% of patients with the disease (Schamroth, 1971). The mechanisms of syncope and sudden death are complex and include asystole (Joseph *et al.*, 1972). The obstructed outflow of the left ventricle is made worse by increased contractility and decreased volume. Arrhythmias (ventricular tachycardia and fibrillation) plus the abnormal haemodynamics contribute to the syncope. Canedo *et al.* (1980) found arrhythmias in 88% of 33 patients with the disease followed for four years. The arrhythmias were life-threatening in 39% and almost all patients had more than one type of arrhythmia. They found that aggressive treatment of the arrhythmias diminished palpitations, pre-syncope and syncope, and appeared to prevent sudden death. Surgery alone does not always prevent syncope, arrhythmias or sudden death (Maron *et al.*, 1978b) but on occasion it does. Therefore, the mechanical aspects must be the more important in some patients.

Goodwin (1964) believed that ventricular fibrillation was the usual cause of death while Braunwald *et al.* (1964) thought that sudden increases in the obstructive element were important contributors to syncope and death.

The inadequate cardiac output during exercise may be compounded by the response to the baroreceptors in the left ventricle wall. These are stimulated by increased ventricular pressure and initiate bradycardia and systemic and splanchnic vasodilatation.

This disease usually produces symptoms before age 40 and dyspnoea is the commonest. Digitalis worsens it while propranolol is helpful (Braunwald *et al.*, 1964).

Atrial myxoma

This is a rare cause of syncope and the syncope, dyspnoea and cardiac murmurs may be related to postural changes.

Myxoma is eight times more common in the left atrium than the right (Medina and Dreifus, 1983). Intermittent mitral or tricuspid valve obstruction is an important clinical clue to its presence.

Mitral Valve Prolapse (MVP)

This is a debatably rare condition more common in young women and it is difficult to know when it accounts for symptoms. The diagnosis depends on a mid- or late-systolic click plus a systolic murmur. The auscultatory abnormalities change, appear and disappear with changes in the patient's posture. Therefore, one must listen to the heart with the patient sitting, supine and after exercise. The heart is not enlarged and blood pressure is normal. Confirmation depends on echocardiographic demonstration of prolapse of the valve or the posterior leaflet during ventricular systole. The clinical presentation may consist of pre-syncopal vertigo, syncope chest pain or discomfort, palpitations and sudden death.

The majority of people with MVP are asymptomatic. A number of arrhythmias have been associated with it, particularly ventricular fibrillation. Rhythm disorders account for the vertigo, syncope and occasional sudden death which can occur in such cases (Swartz *et al.*, 1977).

The other life-threatening complications consist of valvular endocarditis, ruptured chordae tendineae, and possibly cerebral and retinal transient ischaemia. If the last are caused by emboli originating on or near the abnormal valve, it is anomalous that the reports of emboli to other areas (finger-nail beds, flanks, spleen, kidney) are so rare.

Winkle *et al.* (1975) studied 24 patients with MVP by means of exercise testing and 24-h Holter monitoring. A majority of the patients had complex ventricular arrhythmias including ventricular tachycardia. The patients generally were symptom-free during the recorded arrhythmias and normal rhythm was recorded when they complained of palpitations.

DeMaria *et al.* (1974), in a similar study of 20 patients with MVP, found frequent ventricular premature contractions in 40%, sinus tachycardia or atrial premature contractions in 20%, and episodes of abrupt sinus bradycardia, sinus arrest or exaggerated sinus arrhythmia in 30%.

Shappell and Marshall (1975) recognized two distinct groups of patients with the ballooning posterior leaflet syndrome. The first are asymptomatic patients in whom a mid-systolic click, late systolic murmur, or both, and a typical echocardiographic appearance are discovered in the course of an examination for some unrelated symptom.

The second group are those with directly related symptoms, i.e. fatigue, palpitation, chest pain and syncope. These authors suggested that an assessment or precipitation of an arrhythmia should be the first step in investigation. Even when ventricular fibrillation is not provoked by exercise, they recommended drug therapy because of the risk of sudden death. Diphenylhydantoin can shorten a prolonged Q–T interval as can propranolol. They thought that some emotionally-induced event could determine the ventricular fibrillation and there was a contributory central neurogenic mechanism.

Coronary Artery Disease

Syncope occurs with acute and chronic coronary artery disease, with and without chest pain. There are several mechanisms to account for the syncope:

1. An acute episode of myocardial ischaemia can produce sudden pump failure, reduced cardiac output, cerebral perfusion and syncope.
2. More common is a disturbance in rhythm, particularly ventricular tachycardia, or fibrillation and sinus bradycardia. The sinus and AV nodes each have a single coronary artery as a source of blood and are vulnerable to ischaemia with inferior or posterior myocardial infarctions.

Of 308 patients with acute myocardial infarctions, 17% had bradycardia and hypotension and 60% had either syncope or pre-syncopal vertigo (Chadde *et al.*, 1975).

Chiche *et al.* (1974) reported two patients with angina pectoris resulting in syncope. The collapse occurred at the peak of the angina attack and was due to ventricular standstill in one and ventricular tachycardia in the other. Both were relieved of the syncope with a pacemaker.

Ranganathan and Maron (1971) have also described paroxysmal AV block at the time of angina and Harper *et al.* (1975) have described a patient with syncopal episodes, Prinzmetal angina, and transient AV block following an anteroseptal infarction. A pacemaker had no effect on the syncope. It was thought to be due to coronary artery spasm, transient ischaemia of the left ventricle and reduced cardiac output. The angina and its consequences were prevented by coronary artery vasodilator therapy.

Bashour *et al.* (1982) and Beltran *et al.* (1982) have also described sinus node dysfunction and syncope from coronary artery spasm. The patient of Beltran *et al.* had attacks in his sleep, recognized by his wife because the quality of his snoring changed and she then found him unrousable. When he did come around, he was incontinent, stared at the ceiling and was unresponsive for 30 sec.

Irving and Kitchin (1975) reported two patients with syncope associated with severe coronary artery disease and angina on effort. They suggested that the syncopal attacks were secondary to arrhythmias.

Chronic Bifascicular Block

The conduction system of the ventricles consists of three fascicles; the right-bundle branch and the anterior and posterior limbs of the left-bundle branch. Bifascicular block may consist of a block of the right-bundle plus a left-anterior or posterior hemi-block or complete left-bundle branch block.

Dhingra *et al.* (1974) studied prospectively 186 patients with chronic bifascicular block. They were observed for one year. Thirty patients had syncope due to cardiac and non-cardiac causes. The syncope was often benign, not recurrent and was not a predictor of sudden death. It was suggested that permanent pacing was indicated only in those patients with documented serious bradyarrhythmia. Ezri *et al.* (1983) studied 13 patients with chronic bifascicular block and syncope. They found that ventricular tachycardia was a significant cause of syncope in their group.

Syncope After Pacemaker Installation

Alicandri *et al.* (1978) have emphasized the importance of atrial reflexes in a hypothesis explaining episodic hypotension and syncope which may occur after installation of a pace-maker. Their three patients had pacemaker implantation for bradyarrhythmia, and then had attacks of symptomatic hypotension, pre-syncopal vertigo or syncope. Haemodynamic studies revealed a small drop in cardiac output, insufficient to explain the episodic drop in systemic blood pressure.

The periods of activation of the ventricular pacemaker were associated with cannon waves in the right-atrial pressure tracing and these coincided with the drop in systemic blood pressure. External inhibition of the pacemaker was marked by return of sinus rhythm, disappearance of the cannon waves and the fluctuations in blood pressure, and the appearance of a stable blood pressure at a higher level.

The authors suggested that dissociated AV function stimulates two opposing reflexes: the aortic, carotid sinus baroreceptor mechanisms attempting to overcome reduced cardiac output by vasoconstriction, and atrial distention which induces peripheral vasodilatation.

Variations in systemic blood pressure in relationship to the sequence of atrial and ventricular contractions have been reported by Martin and Cobb (1966) but hypotension, pre-syncope, and syncope in ambulatory patients with functioning ventricular pacemakers in place has not previously been described.

The data suggest that the symptoms were due to inappropriate timing of the atrial contraction, increased intra-atrial pressure, peripheral vasodilatation, and then hypotension leading to syncope.

Braunwald *et al.* (1964) have shown that systemic blood pressure is higher in a cardiac cycle in which ventricular contraction is preceded by an appropriately timed atrial systole.

Further support is provided by the work of Kahl *et al.* (1974). They demonstrated that balloon inflation of the left atrium decreased cardiac output and arterial pressure with no compensatory increase in peripheral resistance, while a similar decrease in output from occlusion of the superior vena cava was compensated by a substantial increase in peripheral resistance. Both Alicandri *et al.* (1978) and Kahl *et al.* (1974) suggested that when the atrium contracts against a closed valve, a vasodilatation reflex is established by stimulation of the vagal receptors in the atria and this reflex overcomes the vasoconstriction one would expect from stimulation of the carotid/aortic baroreceptors.

There are other examples of pacemaker failure related to one particular design of pacer. Replacement with a unit of different design relieved the symptoms (Friedberg, 1969).

PATIENT ASSESSMENT

Many patients with an abnormal cardiac rhythm are not aware of it. The methods of assessment, in addition to careful history and physical examination, are ECG, exercise testing, ambulatory monitoring, and electrophysiological studies, as well as a search for extra-cardiac causes.

Resting Electrocardiogram

This has limited value in detection of an intermittent rhythm abnormality. Abnormalities which are known to provoke syncope such as the long QT syndrome (see Chapter 8), myocardial infarction, second- and third-degree AV block can be identified. The significance of isolated ventricular premature beats depends on other cardiac disease(s) present. Sinus bradycardia may be normal in the elderly or well-trained athlete, but may be part of abnormal sinus node function. First- and second-degree AV blocks are not necessarily abnormal and may have no relationship to a syncopal episode (Meytes *et al.*, 1975; Camm *et al.*, 1980; Talan *et al.*, 1982): 'The presence of *high risk* bundle branch blocks on the ECG of a patient evaluated for syncope is usually alarming, but the conduction system disease will progress in only a small percentage of patients and they tend not to suffer from recurrent syncope.' (Dhingra *et al.*, 1974.)

Exercise Testing

This is an attempt to precipitate an arrhythmia and/or syncopal episode by exercising the patient, usually on a treadmill. It is a hospital procedure, must be supervised by a doctor, and requires continual monitoring and the presence of complete resuscitation equipment and a knowledgeable person to use it.

The consensus is that there is a better chance of detecting an intermittent arrhythmia by ambulatory monitoring rather than exercise testing (Boudoulas *et al.*, 1978; Boudoulas *et al.*, 1979; Hartzeanu *et al.*, 1979; Luxon *et al.*, 1980).

Ambulatory Monitoring

A 24-h period of ambulatory monitoring accompanied by the patient's diary of activities during this time may be diagnostic.

However, the relationship between dysrhythmias detected by this means and the patient's symptoms, is not high. A study of 371 monitored patients by Zeldis *et al.* (1980) revealed

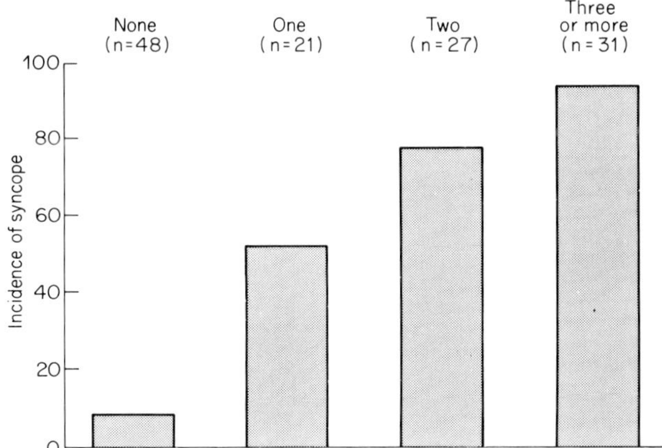

Figure 5.2 The relationship between the number of abnormalities found on electrophysiological studies and the incidence of syncope. (Reproduced by permission of H. Boudoulas *et al.* and the *Journal of Electrocardiology*, 1978, **11**(4): 340.)

that 13% had symptoms and abnormal rhythm at the same time; 34% had their typical symptoms with no rhythm change while 86% recorded tachycardias and remained symptom-free.

Alternatively, hypertropic cardiomyopathy which commonly presents with arrhythmic syncope has a high yield from long-term monitoring. Canedo *et al.* (1980) found 88% of symptomatic patients with this disease had arrhythmias revealed by monitoring.

Electrophysiological Studies

This is a direct, invasive, assessment of the cardiac impulse-generating and conducting system. These studies may be performed when the resting ECG, exercise testing and Holter monitoring have not revealed a diagnosis. They assess in order the sino-atrial node, atria, atrioventricular node, His bundle, and Purkinje system, and may be used to provoke supraventricular and ventricular tachycardias. By this means a pathological tachycardia may be defined and anti-arrhythmic medication tested.

The indications for physiological studies are not clear. In general, they are only for patients with recurrent syncope in whom all other methods of diagnosis have proven fruitless. There is a direct correlation between the likelihood of syncope and the number of abnormalities found on electrophysiological studies (Fig. 5.2). To place the various diagnostic aids in perspective, the following opinion from Boudoulas *et al.* (1982) is a synopsis:

> "In our experience, in patients with no obvious cause of syncope or presyncope, and in whom arrhythmia is strongly suspected, the cause of the symptoms has been detected by ambulatory monitoring alone in approximately 50% by electrophysiologic studies alone in 65–70%, and with exercise testing alone in only 10% of patients."

The success of each of these methods and their combined success rate is shown in Fig. 5.3.

After the usual ECG and general investigations, the next approach should be ambulatory monitoring, then exercise testing and physiological studies last.

Von Leitner and Meyer (1977) assessed 50 patients with pre-syncope or syncope. All had

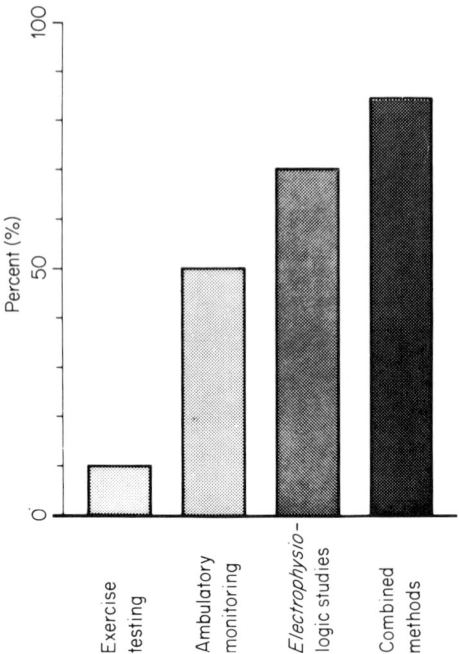

Figure 5.3 The sensitivity of each method of patient assessment alone and combined in the detection of arrhythmia as a cause of syncope. (Reproduced by permission from H. Boudoulas *et al.* (1982) *Current Problems in Cardiology—The Diagnosis of Syncope.* Vol. 7 (ed. H. Boudoulas). p. 33. Chicago: Year Book Medical Publishers.)

stable sinus rhythm without SA node or AV block on routine ECG. Of the 50, only 22% had normal His bundle studies.

Kaul *et al.* (1986) in a study of 15 similar patients established a treatable diagnosis in almost half with electrophysiological studies.

Boudoulas *et al.* (1978) used this method to evaluate 65 patients whose syncope was unexplained by the resting ECG. None had heart disease commonly associated with syncope.

The number of abnormalities on electrophysiological study correlated better with the likelihood of syncope than the severity of any single abnormality. Thus, syncope occurred in 93% of patients with three or more abnormalities, 77% of patients with two abnormalities, 52% of patients with one abnormality and 8% of patients with no abnormalities (Fig. 5.2).

Monitoring and electrophysiological studies can be complementary. Boudoulas *et al.* (1983) in another study of 65 syncopal patients compared the two assessment methods. Patients with an obvious cause of syncope or arrhythmia were excluded. Monitoring was diagnostic in 31 patients and electrophysiological studies were revealing in 42, the combination explaining the symptoms in 51 (78%) patients.

Teichman *et al.* (1985) have assessed electrophysiological studies in syncope of unknown origin in 150 patients prospectively. Syncope of unknown origin (SUO) was defined as syncope or near-syncope unexplained after customary non-invasive evaluation including history, physical examination, routine laboratory screening, EEG, nuclear brain scan, CT

Table 5.4 Synopsis of cardiac syncope

- Cardiac syncope is most commonly due to disordered cardiac rhythm, which may or may not be caused by heart disease
- Abnormalities of cardiac rate and rhythm are common in the asymptomatic public
- The episodic arrhythmias which often cause syncope are the 'sick sinus syndrome', atrioventricular block (second and third degree), complex ventricular dysrhythmias and sino-atrial bradycardia
- Symptoms of these arrhythmias may be brief syncope, extended syncope (1–1.5 h), epilepsy, focal cerebral ischaemic episodes, as well as chest pain, palpitations and dyspnoea
- Aortic stenosis and idiopathic subaortic stenosis cause syncope by obstruction to ventricular outflow, rhythm disturbances and reflex peripheral vasodilatation unaccompanied by adequate increased cardiac output
- Syncope occurs from coronary artery disease with and without angina
- In the assessment of the patient with cardiac syncope, the order of investigations are: history and physical plus routine laboratory screen followed by repeated resting ECG, exercise testing, Holter monitoring and invasive physiological testing. The last three methods in combination yield a higher percentage of diagnoses than any other method alone
- Syncope due to cardiac disease may be followed or accompanied by an epileptic seizure. All idiopathic epileptics with negative EEGs should have a cardiac assessment

scan, 12-lead ECG, chest x-ray, orthostatic vital signs, bed-side carotid sinus massage and 24-h continuous ECG monitoring. Their study included 95 men and 55 women, with a mean age of 62 years.

They found 162 abnormal electrophysiological findings that could explain the SUO in 112 patients, i.e. a diagnostic yield of 75%. One abnormal finding was present in 71 patients, two in 32 patients and three in 9 patients. These were His–Purkinje disease in 49 patients (30%), inducible ventricular arrhythmias in 36 (22%), AV node disease in 20 (12%), sinus node disease in 19 (12%), inducible supraventricular arrhythmias in 18 (11%), carotid sinus hypersensitivity (not elicited by massage prior to electrophysiological studies) in 15 (9%) and hypervagotonia in 5 (3%).

The principal features of cardiac syncope are summarized in Table 5.4.

REFERENCES

Abdon NJ and Malcrona R (1975) High pacemaker implantation rate following 'cardiogenic neurology'. *Acta Medica Scandinavica* **198**: 455–461.

Adelman AG and Wigle ED (1969) The bradycardia, tachycardia, asystole syndrome: treatment by pacemaker. *Canadian Medical Association Journal* **100**: 75–77.

Alicandri C, Fouad FM, Tarazi RC, Castle L and Morant V (1978) Three cases of hypotension and syncope with ventricular pacing: possible role of atrial reflexes. *American Journal of Cardiology* **42**(1): 137–142.

Bashour TT, Hakim O, Ennis AL and Cheng TO (1982) Coronary artery spasm with sinus node dysfunction and syncope. *Archives of Internal Medicine* **142**(9): 1719–1721.

Beltran P, Lichstein E, Sanders M, Hollander G, Greengart A and Jonas S (1982) Coronary artery spasm appearing as syncope. *Archives of Internal Medicine* **142**(1): 192–194.

Birchfield RI, Menefee EE and Bryant GDN (1957) Disease of the sino-atrial node associated with bradycardia, asystole, syncope, and paroxysmal atrial fibrillation. *Circulation* **16**: 20.

Boudoulas H, Schaal SF and Lewis RP (1978) Electrophsiological risk factors of syncope. *Journal of Electrocardiology* **11**(4): 339–342.

Boudoulas H, Dervenagas S, Lewis RP *et al.* (1979) The time course of the blockade of propranolol on sinus node and antrioventricular node. *Journal of Clinical Pharmacology* **19**: 95.

Boudoulas H, Weissler A, Lewis RP and Warren JV (1982) *Current Problems in Cardiology—The Clinical Diagnosis of Syncope*, Vol. 7, No. 7 (ed. H. Boudoulas). pp. 1–40. Chicago: Year Book Medical Publishers.

Boudoulas H, Geleris P, Schaal SF *et al.* (1983) Comparison between electrophysiologic studies and ambulatory monitoring in patients with syncope. *Journal of Electrocardiology* **16**(1): 91–96.

Braunwald E, Lambrew CT, Rockoff SD, Ross J and Morrow AG (1964) Idiopathic hypertrophic subaortic stenosis—a description of the disease based upon an analysis of 64 patients. *Circulation* **3** (**supplement 4**): 3.

Brodsky M, Wu D, Denes P, Kanakis C and Rosen KM (1977) Arrhythmias documented by 24 hour continuous electrocardiographic monitoring in 50 male medical students without apparent heart disease. *American Journal of Cardiology* **29**: 390.

Camm AJ, Evans KE, Ward DE *et al.* (1980) The rhythm of the heart in active elderly subjects. *American Heart Journal* **99**: 598–603.

Canedo MI, Frank MJ and Abdulla AM (1980) Rhythm disturbances in hypertrophic cardiomyopathy: prevalence, relation to symptoms, and management. *American Journal of Cardiology* **45**: 848–855.

Chadde KD, Lichstein E, Gupta PK *et al.* (1975) Bradycardia–hypotension syndrome in acute myocardial infarction: reappraisal of the overdrive effects of atropine. *American Journal of Medicine* **59**: 158–164.

Chiche P, Haiat R and Steff P (1974) Angina pectoris with syncope due to paroxysmal atrioventricular block: role of ischemia. *British Heart Journal* **36**: 577–581.

Clarke JM, Shelton JR, Hamer J, Taylor S and Venning GR (1976) The rhythm of the normal human heart. *Lancet* 2: 508.

DeMaria AN, Amastrdam EA, Vismara LA *et al.* (1974) The variable spectrum of rhythm disturbances in the mitral valve prolapse syndrome. *Circulation* **49–50** (**supplement 111**): 222 (abstract).

Dhingra RC, Denes P, Wu D *et al.* (1974) Syncope in patients with chronic bifascicular block: significance, causative mechanisms, and clinical implications. *Annals of Internal Medicine* **81**: 302-306.

Dreifus LS and Watanabe Y (1971) Localization and significance of atrioventricular block. *American Heart Journal* **82**: 435–438.

Dunning AJ (1979) The cardiac rhythm: normal and abnormal. In *Cerebral Manifestations of Episodic Cardiac Dysrhythmias* (ed. Ewald Busse). Amsterdam and Princeton: Excerpta Medica.

Easley RM and Goldstein S (1971) Sino-atrial syncope. *American Journal of Medicine* **50**(2): 166–167.

Ezri M, Lerman BB, Marchlinski FE, Buxton AE and Josephson ME (1983) Electrophysiologic evaluation of syncope in patients with bifascicular block. *American Heart Journal* **106**(4): 693–697.

Ferrer MI (1968) The sick sinus syndrome in atrial disease. *Journal of the American Medical Association* **206**: 645–646.

Ferrer MI (1973) The sick sinus syndrome. *Circulation* **47**: 635–641.

Fowler NO, Fenton JC and Conway GF (1970) Syncope in cerebral dysfunction caused by bradycardia with atrioventricular block. *American Heart Journal* **80**(3): 303–312.

Friedberg HD (1969) Syncope during stand-by cardiac pacing. *British Heart Journal* **31**: 281–284.

Friedberg CK (1971) Syncope. Pathological physiology: differential diagnosis and treatment (I) and (II). *Modern Concepts of Cardiovascular Disease* **XL**: 55–60, 61–63.

Goodwin JH (1964) Cardiac function in primary myocardial disorders. *British Medical Journal* **1**: 1527.

Hanson JS and Tabakin BS (1965) Comparison of the circulatory responses to upright exercise in 25 'normal' men and 9 distance runners. *British Heart Journal* **27**: 211.

Harper R, Peter T and Hunt D (1975) Syncope in association with Prinzmetal variant angina. *British Heart Journal* **37**: 771–774.

Hartzeanu H, Yahini JH and Neufeld NH (1979) Holter monitoring in dizziness and syncope. *Acta Cardiologica* **34**: 375.

Hinkle LE, Carver ST and Stevens M (1969) The frequency of asymptomatic disturbances of cardiac rhythm and conduction in middle-aged men. *American Journal of Cardiology* **24**: 629–650.

Hiss RG and Lamb LE (1962) Electrocardiographic findings in 122,043 individuals. *Circulation* **25**: 947.

Irving JB and Kitchin AH (1975) Syncopal attacks as symptoms of severe coronary artery disease. *British Medical Journal* **1**: 555–556.

Joseph S, Balcon R and McDonald L (1972) Syncope and hypertrophic obstructive cardiomyopathy due to asystole. *British Heart Journal* **34**: 974–976.

Kahl FR, Flint JF and Szidon JP (1974) Influence of left atrial distension on renal vasomotor tone. *American Journal of Physiology* **226**: 240–246.

Kaul U, Galra GS, Talwark K and Bhatia ML (1986) The value of intracardiac electrophysiologic techniques in recurrent syncope of unknown cause. *International Journal of Cardiology* **10**: 23–31.

Lopez MJ, Runge P, Harrison DC and Schroeder JS (1975) Comparison of 24 versus 12 hours of ambulatory ECG monitoring. *Chest* **67**: 269.

Lown B (1967) Electrical reversion of cardiac arrhythmias. *British Heart Journal* **29**: 469–489.

Lown B, Tykocinski M, Garfein A and Brooks P (1973) Sleep and ventricular premature beats. *Circulation* **48**: 691.

Luxon LM, Crowther A, Harrison MJ *et al.* (1980) Controlled study of 24-hour ambulatory electrocardiographic monitoring in patients with transient neurological symptoms. *Journal of Neurology, Neurosurgery, and Psychiatry* **43**: 37.

Mark AL, Kioschos JM, Abboud FM *et al.* (1973) Abnormal vascular responses to exercise in patients with aortic stenosis. *Journal of Clinical Investigation* **52**: 1138–1146.

Maron BJ, Lipson LC, Roberts EC, Savage DD and Epstein SE (1978a) 'Malignant' hypertrophic cardiomyopathy: identification of a subgroup of families with unusually frequent premature death. *American Journal of Cardiology* **41**: 1133–1140.

Maron BJ, Merrill WH, Freier PA, Kent KN, Epstein SE and Morrow AG (1978b) Long Term clinical course and symptomatic status of patients after operation for hypertrophic subaortic stenosis. *Circulation* **57**: 1205–1213.

Martin RH and Cobb LA (1966) Observations on the effect of atrial systole in man. *Journal of Laboratory and Clinical Medicine* **68**: 224–232.

McAnulty JH, Rahimtoola SH, Murphy E *et al.* (1982) Natural history of 'high risk' bundle branch block: final report of a prospective study. *New England Journal of Medicine* **307**: 137–143.

Medina RP and Dreifus LS (1983) *Current Problems in Cardiology—Syncope,* Vol. 7, No. 6 (ed. W. Proctor Harvey) pp. 1–50. Chicago: Year Book Medical Publishers.

Meytes I, Kaplinsky E, Yahini JH *et al.* (1975) Wenckebach A–V block: a frequent feature following heavy physical training. *American Heart Journal* **90**: 426–430.

Narula OS, Samet P and Javier RP (1972) Significance of the sinus-node recovery time. *Circulation* **45**: 140–158.

Ranganathan N and Maron BJ (1971) Electrocardiographic clues in diagnosing syncope. *Postgraduate Medicine* **49**(3): 126–131.

Ross J and Braunwald E (1968) *Aortic Stenosis.* Circulation **37** (**supplement 5**): 61–67.

Rubenstein JJ, Schulman CL, Yurchak PM and DeSanctis RW (1972) Clinical spectrum of the sick sinus syndrome. *Circulation* **46**: 5–13.

Schamroth L (1971) *The Disorders of Cardiac Rhythm.* p. 238. Oxford and Edinburgh: Blackwell Scientific Publications.

Schwartz LS, Goldfischer J, Sprague GJ and Schwartz SP (1969) Syncope and sudden death in aortic stenosis. *American Journal of Cardiology* **23**(5): 647–658.

Seda PE, McAnulty JH and Anderson CJ (1980) Postural heart block. *British Heart Journal* **44**: 221–223.

Shappell SD and Marshall CE (1975) Ballooning posterior leaflet syndrome. *Archives of Internal Medicine* **135**: 664–667.

Shelton JR (1986) Personal communication. Letter report on follow-up patients reported by Clarke *et al.* (1976).

Shillingford J and Thomas M (1968) Treatment of bradycardia hypotension syndrome in patients with acute myocardial infarction. *American Heart Journal* **75**: 843.

Short DS (1954) Syndrome of alternating bradycardia and tachycardia. *British Heart Journal* **16**: 208–212.

Simonsen E, Straede NJ and Lyager NB (1980) Sinus node dysfunction in 128 patients: a retrospective study with follow-up. *Acta Medica Scandinavica* **208**: 343–348.

Stern S and Tzivoni D (1976) Atrial and ventricular asystole for 19 seconds with syncope. *Israel Journal of Medicine* **12**(1): 28–33.

Sutton R and Perrins EJ (1979) Neurological manifestations of the sick sinus syndrome. In *Cerebral Manifestations of Episodic Cardiac Dysrhythmias* (ed. Ewald Busse) pp. 174–181. Amsterdam and Princeton: Excerpta Medica.

Swartz MH, Teichholz LZE and Donoso E (1977) Mitral valve prolapse, a review of associated arrhythmias. *American Journal of Medicine* **62**: 377–389.

Talan Da, Baurenfeind RA, Ashley WW *et al.* (1982) Twenty-four hour continuous ECG recordings in long-distance runners. *Chest* **82**: 19–24.

Teichman SL, Felder SD, Matas JA, Kim SG, Waspe LE and Fisher JD (1985) The value of electrophysiologic studies in syncope of undetermined origin: report of 150 cases. *American Heart Journal* **110**(2): 469–479.

Von Herbinger W (1961) Gehäufte synkoen bei sino auricularem block. *Cardiologia* **38**: 267.

Von Leitner ER and Meyer V (1977) His electrocardiogram during atrial stimulation in 50 patients with transient cerebral symptoms. *Advances in Cardiology* **19**: 273–276.

Winkle RA, Lopes MG, Fitzgerald JW *et al.* (1975) Arrhythmias in patients with mitral valve prolapse. *Circulation* **52**: 73–81.

Zeldis SM, Levine BJ, Michelson E *et al.* (1980) Cardiovascular complaints: correlation with cardiac arrhythmias on 24-hour electrocardiographic monitoring. *Chest* **78**: 456–462.

6

Autonomic Nervous System Failure

INTRODUCTION

Patients with this disorder are often diagnosed as 'idiopathic orthostatic hypotension' (IOH) because of the pre-eminence of this startling symptom. The defects of sweating, micturition, sexual and bowel function are less or ignored. One of the earliest descriptions of the syndrome was entitled 'postural hypotension' (Bradbury and Eggleston, 1925) and the terms 'idiopathic orthostatic hypotension' and 'progressive autonomic failure' are, to some extent, erroneously used interchangeably. IOH can occur without other neurological disease.

In the past, examples of the syndrome have been labelled by the most obvious symptom because the methods of assessment of the autonomic nervous system have either not been appreciated or not used.

Progressive autonomic failure (PAF) as described by Bannister and Oppenheimer (1982) may be classified into three types:

1. As part of the central, multisystem atrophies (MSA) (Shy–Drager syndrome, Parkinsonism, olivopontocerebellar atrophy) as well as diseases like tabes dorsalis and syringomyelia.
2. As part of some peripheral nervous system diseases including diabetic, alcoholic, and other neuropathies, as well as familial dysautonomia, the Riley–Day syndrome.
3. Idiopathic orthostatic hypotension alone, not part of either a central or peripheral disease of the nervous system.

In both MSA and IOH, plasma levels of norepinephrine do not increase normally on standing (Ziegler *et al.*, 1977). Patients with IOH have low plasma norepinephrine levels when reclining while patients with MSA have normal basal levels.

As sensitivity to sympathomimetic amines is altered when sympathetic nerves are damaged, responses to drugs may be useful in distinguishing IOH and MSA. Denervation enhances sensitivity to directly acting drugs, but with complete denervation there is no effect of indirectly-acting sympathomimetic agents. Decreased α-adrenergic with normal β-adrenergic responses may be the basis of IOH.

A general classification of autonomic failure is reproduced from Bannister (1983) in Table 6.1

Table 6.1 A classification of autonomic failure. (Reproduced with permission from OUP, *Autonomic Failure*, 1983, ed. Sir Roger Bannister. Oxford: Oxford University Press.)

1. Primary
   - (a) Progressive autonomic failure (PAF) (Bradbury and Eggleston, 1925)
   - (b) Progressive autonomic failure with multiple system atrophy (MSA) (Shy and Drager, 1960)
   - (c) Progressive autonomic failure with Parkinson's disease (PD) (Fichefet *et al.*, 1965).
2. Secondary
   - (a) General medical disorders; diabetes (Low *et al.*, 1975a)
   - (b) Autoimune disease; acute and subacute dysautonomia (Young *et al.*, 1969; Hopkins *et al.*, 1974); Guillain–Barré syndrome; myasthaenia (Maclean and Horton, 1937); rheumatoid arthritis (Edmunds *et al.*, 1979)
   - (c) Carcinomatous autonomic neuropathy (Park *et al.*, 1972)
   - (d) Metabolic diseases; porphyria (Shirger *et al.*, 1962); Tangier disease, inherited (recessive) α-lipoprotein deficiency; Fabry's disease
   - (e) Hereditary sensory neuropathies, dominant or recessive (Dyck and Ohta, 1975)
   - (f) Infections of the nervous system; syphilis, Chagas' disease
   - (g) Central brain lesions; vascular lesions or tumours involving the hypothalamus and the midbrain, for example, craniopharyngioma (Thomas *et al.*, 1961)
   - (h) Spinal cord lesions
   - (i) Familial dysautonomia
   - (j) Familial hyperbradykinism (Streeten *et al.*, 1972)
3. Drugs
   - (i) Selective neurotoxic drugs (Le Quesne, 1975): alcoholism (Low *et al.*, 1975b); Wernicke's encephalopathy (Gravallese and Victor, 1957)
   - (ii) Tranquillizers: phenothiazines, barbiturates
   - (iii) Antidepressants: tricyclics (Glassman *et al.*, 1979); monoamine oxidase inhibitors
   - (iv) Vasodilator hypotensive drugs: prazocin, hydrallazine
   - (v) Centrally acting hypotensive drugs: methyldopa, clonidine
   - (vi) Adrenergic neuron blocking drugs: guanethidine, bethanidine, debroisoquin
   - (vii) α-Adrenergic blocking drugs: phenoxybenzamine, labetolol
   - (viii) Ganglion-blocking drugs: hexamethonium, mecamylamine
   - (ix) Angiotensin converting enzyme inhibitors: captopril

CLINICAL FEATURES

The clinical aspects of autonomic failure are similar irrespective of the aetiology. Orthostatic syncope alone is equally common in the two sexes, but autonomic failure as part of multisystem atrophy is twice as common in men, usually occurring in middle age, and is more common with advancing age. Orthostatic hypotension in association with peripheral nerve disease has a clearly different pathogenesis than the same symptom occurring as part of multisystem atrophy. The latter has protean manifestations, one of which is a failure to regulate an **intact** peripheral autonomic system.

The essential common symptom irrespective of the site of the lesion is lightheadedness, a feeling of being about to faint, or fainting on standing with relief on sitting or lying down. In retrospect, this is often not the first symptom but it almost inevitably takes the patient to the doctor while the other common complaints of failing libido, impotence, urinary incontinence and frequency are more readily accepted as 'normal' considering the age of the average patient. Caird *et al.* (1973), in a study on the effect of posture on blood pressure in the normal elderly, found that the systolic pressure after standing fell by 20 mmHg in 24% of subjects, 36 mmHg or more in 9% and 40 mmHg more in 5%. There was no sex difference but the larger drop in systolic pressure was much more common in those over 75 years of age.

The syncopal sensations on standing progress slowly over seconds and minutes and usually allow the patient to sit down or lie down before collapse. The retarded tempo is a clear differentiating factor from the crashing abruptness of the 'drop attack' and Adams–Stokes attack, also seen in patients of this age. Bannister (1983) and Polinsky (1984) both noted the aching pain in the neck, shoulders and occiput, felt just before consciousness is lost.

Some patients with autonomic failure may tolerate a systolic blood pressure (standing) of 60–75 mmHg with no symptoms. Apparently cerebral autoregulation is functional but at levels 20–30 mmHg below the point at which it would fail in normal subjects (Thomas and Bannister, 1981).

At the start of the syncope there may be other hints of basilar artery distribution ischaemia in the form of visual obscurations, formed objects in the vision, circumoral paraesthesiae and hiccoughs. An alert witness will report details unlike the situation in a vasovagal faint. The patient does not sweat, the pulse does not slow, and the grey-white pallor of an asystolic faint is not as obvious.

Inquiry reveals that some or all of the following make the symptoms more frequent and more severe:

- a period of enforced bed rest for any cause, i.e. influenza, a fractured hip
- drinking alcohol, eating a big meal
- in the early part of the day
- after exercise
- during hot weather
- a combination of the above, i.e. while standing after breakfast

Further history-taking confirms the absence of sweating and in the male, loss of libido and potency. Bladder symptoms are common in both sexes including frequency, urgency, nocturia, as well as incomplete emptying and retention. (When autonomic failure is part of the more diffuse multisystem diseases, some of which have upper motor neurone lesions, the bladder symptoms and malfunctions have more than a single cause.)

The common bowel complaint is severe and progressive constipation, often leading to rectal incontinence.

PATIENT ASSESSMENT

The following concerns only the assessment of autonomic function. The other manifestations of diseases (Shy–Drager, Parkinsonism) which may have autonomic nervous system involvement are outside the scope of this chapter.

Table 6.2 from Bannister (1983) shows some of the tests which may reveal whether a

Table 6.2 Some tests of autonomic function. (Reproduced with permission from OUP *Autonomic Failure*, 1983, ed. Sir Roger Bannister. Oxford: Oxford University Press.)

1. Sympathetic efferent constrictor fibres to capacity and resistance vessels:
   (a) Postural hypotension
   (b) Lack of overshoot after Valsalva test
   (c) Lack of blood pressure rise on stress
   (d) Low resting plasma noradrenaline
   (e) Lack of rise of plasma noradrenaline on tilting
2. Sympathetic efferent fibres to heart:
   (a) Lack of tachycardia during Valsalva, phase II
   (b) Lack of tachycardia on tilting
   (c) Lack of tachycardia on cortical arousal
   (d) Lack of tachycardia on isometric exercise
2. Parasympathetic efferent fibres to heart:
   (a) Lack of sinus arrhythmia
   (b) Lack of effect of carotid massage
   (c) Lack of rise of cardiac rate with atropine

patient with autonomic neuropathy has a sympathetic efferent defect to blood vessels or a sympathetic or parasympathetic lesion to the heart. Only some of these are discussed.

Blood Pressure and Posture

The most important factor determining blood pressure, under basal conditions, is the resistance of the arterial tree. The rate and stroke volume of the heart, while important, are secondary. The constriction and therefore resistance of arteries is a compromise between the functions of the pressor and depressor areas of the medullary cardiovascular centres plus local environmental factors. The inhibitory and to a lesser extent excitatory peripheral stimuli maintaining normal blood pressure are conveyed from carotid, aortic and other baroreceptors, the first probably being the most important.

The patient with orthostatic hypotension must have his blood pressure taken supine after resting for 15 minutes and then on standing. Blood pressure is taken immediately and after 3–5 min of standing. A slow baroreceptor response does not necessarily mean autonomic failure. A fall in systolic pressure of more than 30 mmHg in the standing position is abnormal and warrants further investigation.

There are several other bedside assessments of the autonomic nervous system as follows.

Valsalva Manoeuvre

This is a relatively easy test of sympathetic efferent fibres to vessels and of sympathetic and parasympathetic fibres to the heart. It can be performed at the bedside, requires a continuous ECG tracing, and is invalid with an uncooperative patient.

With the patient sitting, midway in the respiratory cycle, he must blow into a closed system maintaining a pressure of 50 mmHg for 15–20 sec. Blowing into the rubber tubing connected to the mercury-containing reservoir and glass column of a sphygmomanometer is a practical method. The normal negative intrathoracic pressure becomes positive,

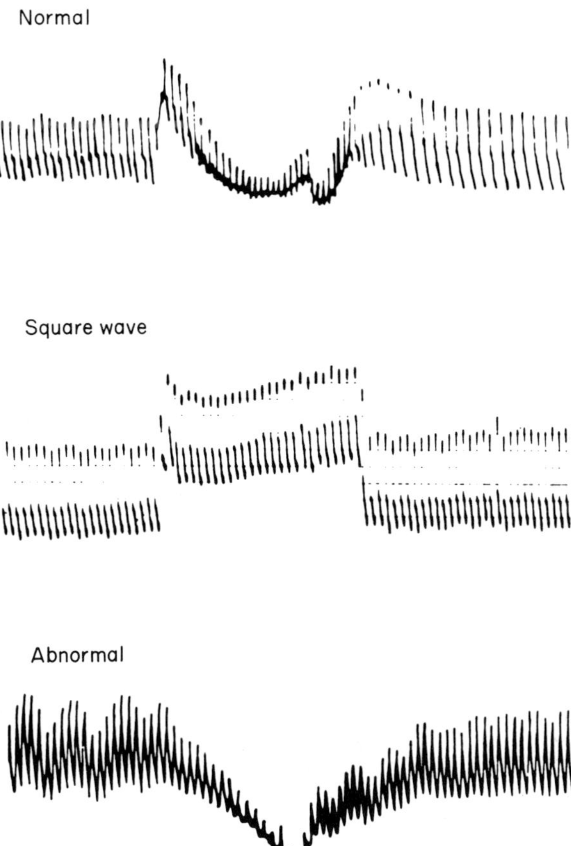

Figure 6.1 Intra-arterial blood pressure recording during valsalva manoeuvre. The upper trace is normal. The middle trace 'square-wave' is found in heart failure where the baroreceptors do not respond. The lower trace is from an autonomic neuropathy. There is no evidence of circulatory reflexes as blood pressure falls throughout the strain, recovers slowly with no overshoot and the pulse is unchanged. (Modified from Sharpey-Schafer (1965), and Johnson and Spalding (1974), and reproduced with permission from OUP, *Autonomic Failure*, 1983, ed. Sir Roger Bannister. Oxford: Oxford University Press.)

central venous return is impeded, and changes in blood pressure with inverse changes in pulse rate occur. The normal intra-arterial blood pressure and pulse changes are shown in Fig. 6.1.

At the start of straining, Phase 1 is a short (seconds) increase in blood pressure with decrease in heart rate; Phase 2 is a decrease in blood pressure and increasing pulse rate as straining continues; Phase 3 after release of strain is a short (seconds) further fall in blood pressure while the pulse continues to accelerate; Phase 4 is an upward rebound in blood pressure and a marked bradycardia.

The valsalva ratio (Levin, 1966) is the longest R–R interval (bradycardia) after the test to the shortest interval during the test. Bennett *et al.* (1978) consider a ratio of 1.21 or greater as normal, 1.11–1.20 as borderline, and 1.10 or less as abnormal (Ewing, 1983).

Heart Rate Changes

The normal heart beat is irregular and this 'respiratory sinus arrhythmia' is dependent on efferent parasympathetic function. It vanishes in diabetics, presumably as part of an autonomic neuropathy.

Natelson (1985) has described a method of recording the low frequency pulse variations which are not visible to the naked eye as changing R–R intervals. These variables are influenced by both sides of the autonomic nervous system and hormonal factors (Akselrod *et al.*, 1981). The method is spectral analysis which breaks up the pulse rate into each of its recurrent frequencies (Fig. 6.2). The differences in the proportions of pulse frequencies between normal, moderate diabetics and diabetics with orthostatic hypotension are striking.

Respiration

Respiratory sinus arrhythmia is an increase in pulse rate with inspiration and a decrease with expiration and is mediated entirely by the phasic activity of the vagus nerves. It is abolished by vagal section or atropine, persists if breathing is paralyzed, and is unaffected by propranolol. It is a function of parasympathetic control of the heart rate (Wheeler and Watkins, 1973; Ewing, 1978; Ewing *et al.*, 1980).

The easiest method of measurement is continuous ECG recording while the subject breathes deeply in and out at 6 breaths/minute. Ewing (1983) has suggested that differences in rate of 15/min or more are normal, 11–14/min borderline, and 10/min or less are abnormal. An abnormal result indicates a parasympathetic neuropathy. The test is not applicable if the subject does not have sinus rhythm.

Postural Change

The normal subject has an immediate tachycardia on changing from the supine to the upright. The R–R shortening is maximum at about the 15th beat after standing. There is then a relative bradycardia, maximum at about the 30th beat after standing. Ewing (1978) has demonstrated the absence of these changes in diabetics with autonomic neuropathy. He has designated the R–R interval at the 30th and 15th beats as the 30:15 ratio, normal being 1.04 or greater while 1.00 or less is abnormal.

Sustained Hand Grip

In the normal an isometric exercise-like-sustained hand grip will be accompanied by an increase in systemic blood pressure. This is due initially to a heart-rate-dependent increase in cardiac output. Subsequently, sympathetic vasoconstrictor fibres and increased peripheral resistance will contribute to the elevation of blood pressure.

Ewing (1983) has defined a rise of diastolic blood pressure of 15 mmHg or more, on maximum voluntary contraction of a hand grip dynamometer as normal, 11–15 mmHg as borderline, and 10 mmHg or less as indicative of autonomic damage in particular to sympathetic efferent pathways.

The normal values and range of responses for these tests are shown in Table 6.3 In addi-

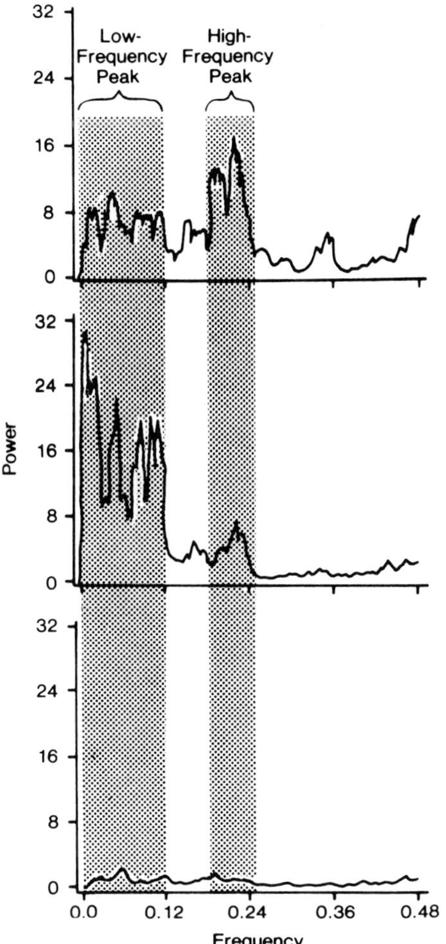

Figure 6.2 A continuous 10-min power spectral analysis of pulse frequencies (R–R intervals) digitized from a standard ECG. The top panel is from a normal subject, middle panel a diabetic and bottom panel a severe diabetic with orthostatic hypotension. The patient in the bottom panel has no evidence of significant autonomic efferents to the heart. (Reproduced with permission from B. H. Natelson and *Archives of Neurology*, 1985, **42**: 178–184.)

tion, their relative sensitivity is shown in Fig. 6.3 where they have been applied to 288 diabetics.

Cold Pressor Test and Others

Placing one hand in 4°C water raises the blood pressure in the other arm and reduces finger blood flow. The afferent components of this reflex are the spino-thalamic system, and peripheral pain/temperature conducting fibres. It is an inappropriate test for autonomic assessment in diabetics whose peripheral sensation is often severely abnormal and in excess of their symptoms (Moorhouse and Chochinov, 1972). The efferent side is sympathetic and

Table 6.3 The normal values and range of responses for some simple means of assessing cardiovascular reflexes. (Reproduced with permission from D. J. Ewing and OUP, in *Autonomic Failure*, 1983, ed. Sir Roger Bannister. Oxford: Oxford University Press.)

	Normal	Borderline	Abnormal
1. Valsalva manoeuvre (Valsalva ratio)	1.21 or more	1.11–1.20	1.10 or less
2. Heart-rate variation (maximum–minimum heart rate)	15 beats/min or more	11–14 beat/min	10 beats/min or less
3. Heart-rate response to standing (30:15 ratio)	1.04 or more	1.01–1.03	1.00 or less
4. Postural fall in blood pressure (fall in systolic BP)	10 mmHg or less	11–29 mmHg	30 mmHg or more
5. Sustained handgrip (increase in diastolic BP)	16 mmHg or more	11–15 mmHg	10 mmHg or less

vasoconstrictor. Hines and Brown (1936) described an average rise of 11 mmHg in normal subjects although some normal subjects had no response. However, the test is helpful when there is a positive cold pressor response and the valsalva manoeuvre is abnormal suggesting an afferent baroreceptor lesion.

The rise in blood pressure in response to mental arithmetic, startle, and loud noises does

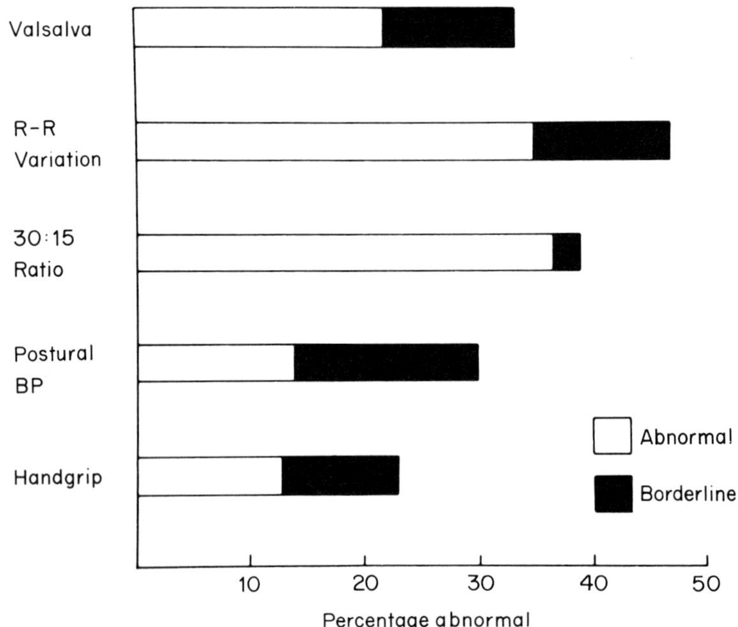

Figure 6.3 The abnormal and borderline responses to the five tests of cardiovascular reflexes used in testing 288 diabetics. (Reproduced with permission from D. J. Ewing in *Autonomic Failure*, 1983, ed. Sir Roger Bannister. Oxford: Oxford University Press.)

not appear to have immediate application to the assessment of autonomic nervous system integrity.

Sweating is usually not investigated in patients with autonomic failure. Bladder and bowel function are usually assessed historically although Bradley (1980) has investigated bladder abnormalities of diabetics.

BIOCHEMISTRY AND PHARMACOLOGY

Epinephrine and Norepinephrine

Norepinephrine (NE) is produced by stimulation of the sympathetic nervous system. NE and epinephrine (E) are produced from stimulation of the adrenal medulla. Noradrenaline levels may be increased by postural change, age, emotion, bleeding, and hypoglycaemia, and diminished by the rate of re-uptake by sympathetic nerve endings.

Plasma noradrenaline levels in patients with multiple system atrophy are normal at rest, while they are lower in patients with IOH alone. Both groups of patients have an exaggerated sensitivity to infused norepinephrine. The assessment of these agents, their precursors, formation, uptake, and metabolites offers a source of information about chronic autonomic failure.

Resting blood pressure, plasma norepinephrine, and epinephrine, are significantly lower in quadriplegics than in normal controls. This may reflect diminshed resting sympathetic nervous activity (Mathias *et al.*, 1976). Golstein *et al.* (1983) have presented evidence that venous plasma norepinephrine provides a reasonable indirect index of sympathetic neural activity. Kopin *et al.* (1983) have differentiated multiple system atrophy patients from idiopathic orthostatic hypotension patients by measurement of urinary catecholamine metabolites, while Polinsky *et al.* (1984) have measured the metabolite 3-methoxy-4-hydroxyphenylglycol (MHPG) in CSF and plasma of patients with chronic autonomic failure. MHPG is the major metabolite of norepinephrine. CSF levels of MHPG are lower in both MSA and IOH patients but only IOH patients have low plasma levels. They concluded that abnormally-functioning central noradrenergic pathways cause the low CSF levels, while in IOH the decreased CSF levels resulted from the diminished plasma MHPG levels.

Polinsky (1983) has defined three separate pharmacologically-distinct groups of patients with orthostatic hypotension. He has used the responses to the pressor agents tyramine, norepinephrine and angiotensin II, as well as the responses of glucose, catecholamines, glucagon, growth hormone, cortisol and pancreatic polypeptide to insulin-induced hypoglycaemia.

Non-traumatic Spinal Cord Disease and Postural Hypotension

Aminoff and Wilcox (1972) reported a 50-year-old patient with syringomyelia and autonomic dysfunction. Her symptoms were orthostatic hypotension, lack of sweating, and bladder and bowel incontinence. On changing from the supine to upright, blood pressure fell from 115/70 to 80/40 with no change in pulse. She was found to have impairment of circulatory reflexes and thermal regulatory sweating and 'systolic' bladder. Autonomic afferent fibres and sympathetic pre- and post-ganglionic fibre integrity were demonstrated. This suggested that the autonomic nervous system was affected at an intermediate point, such as at the foramen magnum, with an interruption of descending autonomic fibres above the syrinx and the upper cervical cord. Clinical assessment indicated that the patient had a syrinx extending from the second and fourth cervical to the eighth thoracic segment and presumably this involved the descending autonomic pathways. The intermediolateral columns or autonomic outflow paths in the spinal cord may also have been affected.

Kennedy and Duchen (1985) have studied quantitatively the intermediolateral column cells in motor neurone disease and the Shy–Drager syndrome. The intermediolateral column neurones in the thoracic spinal cord were counted in five patients who had died of motor neurone disease, two of Shy–Drager syndrome, and three of other neurological diseases not affecting the spinal cord or roots. The number of intermediolateral column cells in all motor neurone disease cases was slightly but not significantly reduced compared to the control cords. By contrast, in Shy–Drager cases there was a highly significant reduction in intermediolateral column cells compared with the normal cords.

Alcoholism

Postural hypotension is common in Wernicke's encephalopathy, probably the result of impaired sympathetic outflow at central or peripheral levels (Victor *et al.*, 1971). However, it is not a common feature of uncomplicated alcohol neuropathy. Novak and Victor (1974) have examined the sympathetic nervous system in three patients with hepatic encephalopathy, Wernicke's disease and severe neuropathy. They found varying degrees of degeneration of the vagus nerve manifest clinically by dysphonia and dysphagia. Their patients has urinary retention or bladder and bowel incontinence as well as hypotension and bradycardia. They concluded that the peripheral neuropathic changes were identical to those of beri-beri. Low *et al.* (1975b) have also performed clinical and pathological studies on the sympathetic nervous system in alcohol neuropathy. Of the 12 subjects with alcohol neuropathy examined, abnormal sweat patterns occurred in all and an abnormal valsalva ratio in one-fifth. Postural hypotension and denervation hypersensitivity were absent in all patients examined. Quantitative assessment of baroreceptor function revealed no abnormalities. Quantitative histological studies of the greater splanchnic nerves in four subjects revealed fibre density within the control range.

TREATMENT

There are several aspects to the treatment of orthostatic hypotension. If the patient is to remain mobile, the orthostatic syncope has to be dealt with. If the defective baroreceptor reflexes are the cause of the orthostatic syncope, the same defect may allow recumbent **hypertension**. When such a patient moves from supine to upright the change in blood pressure may be great enough to provoke local cerebral ischaemic symptoms. Similarly, while recumbent the hypertension may lead to its own complications of cerebral oedema, focal haemorrhage, and papilloedema, etc.

Support Garments

Elastic, hip, or waist high stockings may help (Sheps, 1976). The improvement seems to be

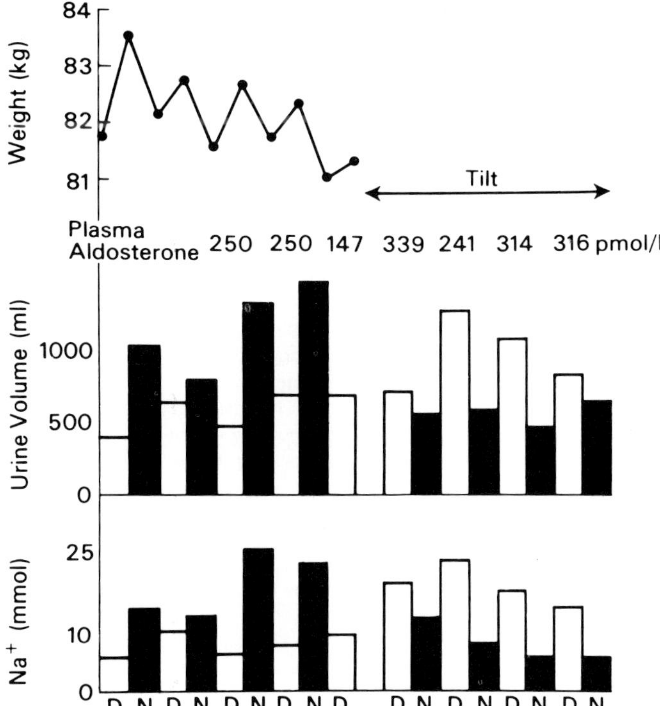

Figure 6.4 Diurnal changes in urine volume and sodium in a patient with multiple system atrophy for 5 days of sleeping flat at night and 5 days of sleeping with head-up tilt. D = daytime, N = night. (Reproduced with permission from OUP, *Autonomic Failure*, 1983, ed. Sir Roger Bannister. Oxford: Oxford University Press.)

short-lived and few patients persist in using these garments. Some patients have had good results with G-suits and are able to tolerate them.

Sleep Position

Plasma volume will increase as will standing and lying blood pressure as the result of sleeping in the sitting position (Maclean and Allen, 1940; Bannister *et al.*, 1969).

A similar improvement can be produced by having the patient sleep with head-up tilt and the day versus night excretion of water and sodium, urine volume and weight (reflecting the increase in extracellular fluid) are shown in Fig. 6.4 This relatively simple night-time change may effectively correct the postural hypotension for several years.

The probable mechanism is reduced renal arterial pressure, increased renin release with angiotension II- and aldosterone-enhanced plasma volume.

Drugs

Fludrocortisone is the nearest to an ideal drug for the treatment of PAF. It increases the

Table 6.4 Various pharmacological agents which may be useful in the treatment of orthostatic hypotension. (Reproduced with permission from R. J. Polinsky, 1984, 'Multiple system atrophy', *Neurologic Clinics,* **2**(3). Philadelphia: W. B. Saunders Co.)

Drugs*	Possible mechanisms of action
Fludrocortisone (A,b,m)	a. Increase sodium and fluid retention
Indomethacin (a,b,g,H)	b. Sensitization of vascular alpha-adrenergic receptors
Propranolol (f,I)	c. Ganglionic stimulation
Pindolol (i,J)	d. Indirectly acting sympathomimetic drug
Ephedrine (D,e)	e. Alpha-agonist drug
Phenylephrine (E)	f. Blockade of neuronal uptake
Mianserin (f,G)	g. Block presynaptic inhibitory adrenergic receptor
Amphetamine (D,e,n)	h. Decrease circulating vasodilator prostaglandins
Methylphenidate (e,N)	i. Inhibit beta-adrenergic activity
MAO inhibitors (O)†	j. Beta-blocker with intrinsic sympathomimetic activity
L-threo-DOPS (K)	k. Increase norepinephrine synthesis
Dihydroergotamine (L)	l. Nonadrenergic vasoconstrictor
Midodrine (E)	m. Inhibits extraneuronal catecholamine uptake
Vasopressin (L)	n. CNS 'stimulant' drug
Caffeine (C,n)	o. Diminish norepinephrine catabolism
Metoclopramide (P)	p. Blocks dopamine receptors
Clonidine (E)	
Yohimbine (G)	
Prednisone (A,b,m)	

* Mechanism of action is shown in parentheses; the primary mechanism is capitalized for those medications with complex actions.
† MAO = monoamine oxidase.

vascular responsiveness to noradrenaline, raises blood pressure in the upright position and expands plasma volume.

The list of drugs in the treatment of orthostatic hypotension is shown in Table 6.4 from Polinsky (1984). Their methods of action suggests the disease has multipe abnormal sites and no one best therapy.

Hoeldtke *et al.* (1986) have used a somatostatin analogue (SMS-201-995) in the treatment of autonomic neuropathy, particularly for the post-prandial hypotension. It proved effective

Table 6.5 Synopsis of autonomic nervous system failure.

- Orthostatic hypotension is the commonest symptom of autonomic nervous system failure
- It may be an isolated symptom of idiopathic origin (IOH) or part of a central nervous system disease, or part of a peripheral nervous system disease
- The autonomic nervous system may be assessed at the bed-side by measurement of the supine and then standing pulse and blood pressure. Also, the pulse and blood-pressure responses to the valsalva manoeuvre, sustained hand grip, cold pressor test and deep breathing are informative
- A large number of drugs have been advocated for the treatment of this disease(s) as well as sleeping in a head-up tilt position

and relieved the hypotension after meals in two of their eight patients who had become refractory to mineralocorticoids, indomethacin and caffeine.

The features of syncope occurring in autonomic nervous system failure are summarized in Table 6.5.

REFERENCES

Akselrod S, Gordon D, Ubel FA *et al.* (1981) Power spectrum analysis of the heart rate fluctuations: a quantitative probe of beat to beat cardiovascular control. *Science* **213**: 220–222.

Aminoff MJ and Wilcox CS (1972) Autonomic dysfunction in syringomyelia. *Postgraduate Medical Journal* **48**: 113–115.

Bannister R (1983) *Autonomic Failure*, p.67. Oxford: Oxford University Press.

Bannister R, Ardill L and Fentem P (1969) An assessment of various methods of treatment of idiopathic hypotension. *Quarterly Journal of Medicine* **38**: 377–395.

Bannister R and Oppenheimer DR (1982) Parkinsonism, system degenerations, and autonomic failure. In *Movement Disorders*, Vol. 2 (Neurology Series) (eds D Marsden and S Fahn). London: Butterworth.

Bennett T, Farquhar IK, Hosking DJ and Hampton JR (1978) Assessment of methods for estimating autonomic nervous control of the heart in patients with diabetes mellitus. *Diabetes* **27**: 1167–1174.

Bradbury S and Eggelston C (1925) Postural hypotension: a report of three cases. *American Heart Journal* **1**: 73–86.

Bradley WE (1980) Diagnosis of urinary bladder dysfunction in diabetes mellitus. *Annals of Internal Medicine* **92**: 323–326.

Caird FI, Andrews GR and Kennedy RD (1973) Effect of posture on blood pressure in the elderly. *British Heart Journal* **35**: 527–530.

Dyck P and Ohta M (1975) Neuronal atrophy and degeneration predominantly affecting peripheral sensory neurons. In *Peripheral Neuropathy*, Vol. 2 (eds PJ Dyck, PK Thomas and EH Lambert) pp. 791–824. Philadelphia: W.B. Saunders.

Edmunds ME, Jones TC, Saunders WA and Sturrock RD (1979) Autonomic neuropathy in rheumatoid arthritis. *British Medical Journal* **2**: 173–175.

Ewing DJ (1978) Cardiovascular reflexes and autonomic neuropathy. *Clinical Science Molecular Medicine* **55**: 321–327.

Ewing DJ (1983). In *Autonomic Failure* (ed. R Bannister), p. 374. Oxford: Oxford University Press.

Ewing DJ, Hume L, Campbell IW, Murray A, Neilson JMM and Clarke BF (1980) Autonomic mechanisms in the intitial heart rate response to standing. *Journal of Applied Physiology* **49**: 809–814.

Fichefet JP, Sternon JE, Franklen L, Demanet JC and Vanderhagen JJ (1965) Étude anatomo-clinique d'un cas d'hypotension orthostatique 'idiopathique.' Considérations pathogenique. *Acta Cardiologica* **20**: 332–348.

Glassman AH, Bigger JT, Giardina EV, Kantor SJ, Perel JM and Davies M (1979) Clinical characteristics of imipramine-induced orthostatic hypotension. *Lancet* **1**: 468–472.

Goldstein DS, McCarty R, Polinsky RJ and Kopin IJ (1983) Relationship between plasma norepinephrine and sympathetic neural activity. *Hypertension* **5**(4): 552–559.

Gravallese MA Jr and Victor M (1957) Circulatory studies on Wernicke's encephalopathy, with special reference to the occurrence of a state of high cardiac output and postural hypotension. *Circulation* **15**: 836–844.

Hines EA and Brown GE (1936) The cold pressor test for measuring the reactibility of the blood pressure. *American Heart Journal* **11**: 1–9.

Hoeldtke RD, O'Dorisio TM and Boden G (1986) Treatment of autonomic neuropathy with a somatostatin analogue SMS-201-995. *Lancet* **2**: 602–605.

Hopkins A, Neville B and Bannister R (1974) Autonomic neuropathy of acute onset. *Lancet* **1**: 769–771.

Kennedy PGE and Duchen LW (1985) A quantitative study of intermediolateral column cells in motor neurone disease and the Shy–Drager syndrome. *Journal of Neurology, Neurosurgery and Psychiatry* **48**: 1103–1106.

Kopin IJ, Polinsky RJ, Oliver JA, Oddershede IP and Ebert MH (1983) Urinary catecholamine metabolites distinguish different types of sympathetic neuronal dysfunction in patients with orthostatic hypotension. *Journal of Clinical Endocrinology and Metabolism* **57**(3): 632–657.

Levin AB (1966) A simple test of cardiac function based upon the heart rate changes induced by the valsalva manoeuver. *American Journal of Cardiology* **18**: 90–99.

Low PA, Walsh JC, Huang CY and McLeod JG (1975a) The sympathetic nervous system in diabetic neuropathy. *Brain* **98**: 341–356.

Low PA, Walsh JC, Huang CY and McLeod JG (1975b) The sympathetic nervous system in a alcoholic neuropathy: a clinical and pathological study. *Brain* **98**: 357–364.

Low PA, Thomas JE and Dyck PJ (1978) The splanchnic autonomic outflow in Shy–Drager syndrome and idiopathic orthostatic hypotension. *Annals of Neurology* **4**: 511–514.

Maclean AR and Horton BT (1937) Myasthenia gravis with postural hypotension. *Proceedings of Staff Meeting Mayo Clinic* **12**: 787.

Maclean AR and Allen EV (1940) Orthostatic hypotension and orthostatic tachycardia. Treatment with the 'head-up' bed. *Journal of the American Medical Association* **115**(25): 2162–2166.

Mathias CJ, Christensen NJ, Corbett JL, Frankel HL and Spalding JMK (1976) Plasma catecholamines during paroxysmal neurogenic hypertension in quadriplegic man. *Circluation Research* **39**: 204–208.

Moorhouse JA and Chochinov RH (1972) Sensory perception thresholds in patients with juvenile diabetes and their close relatives. *New England Journal of Medicine* **286**: 1233–1237.

Natelson BH (1985) Neurocardiology—an interdisciplinary area for the 80's. *Archives of Neurology* **42**: 178–184.

Novak DJ and Victor M (1974) The vagues and sympathetic nerves in alcoholic neuropathy. *Archives of Neurology (Chicago)* **30**: 273–284.

Park DM, Johnson RH, Crean GP and Robinson JF (1972) Orthostatic hypotension with recovery after radiotherapy in a patient with bronchial carcinoma. *British Medical Journal* **3**: 510–511.

Polinsky RJ (1983). In *Autonomic Failure* (ed. R Bannister) pp. 201–236. Oxford: Oxford University Press.

Polinsky RJ (1984) Multiple system atrophy. *Neurologic Clinics* **2**(3): 487–498.

Polinsky RJ, Jimerson DC and Kopin IJ (1984) Chronic autonomic failure, CSF, and plasma 3-methoxy-4-hydroxyphenylglycol. *Neurology (Cleveland)* **34**(7): 979–983.

Sheps SG (1976) The use of an elastic garment in the treatment of idiopathic orthostatic hypotension. *Cardiology* **61**: (**supplement 1**): 271–279.

Shirger A, Martin WJ, Goldstein NP and Huizenga KA (1962) Orthostatic hypotension in association with acute exacerbation of porphyria. *Proceedings of Staff Meeting Mayo Clinic* **37**: 7–11.

Shy GM and Drager GA (1960) A neurological syndrome associated with orthostatic hypotension. *Archives of Neurology (Chicago)* **2**: 511–527.

Streeten DHP, Kerr LP, Kerr CB, Prior JC and Dalakos TG (1972) Hyperbradykininism: a new orthostatic syndrome. *Lancet* **2**: 1048–1053.

Thomas DJ and Bannister R (1980) Preservation of autoregulation of cerebral blood flow in autonomic failure. *Journal of Neurological Sciences* **44**: 205–212.

Thomas JE, Schirger A, Fealey RD and Sheps SG (1981) Orthostatic hypotension. *Proceedings of Staff Meeting Mayo Clinic* **56**: 117–125.

Victor M, Adams RD and Collins GH (1971) *The Wernicke–Korsakoff Syndrome*. Philadelphia: F.A. Davies.

Wheeler T and Watkins PJ (1973) Cardiac denervation in diabetes. *British Medical Journal* **4**: 584–586.

Young RR, Asbury AK, Adams RD and Corbett JL (1969) Pure pan-dysautonomia with recovery. *Transactions of the American Neurological Association* **94**: 355–357.

Ziegler MC, Lake CR and Kopin IJ (1977) The sympathetic nervous system defect in primary orthostatic hypotension. *New England Journal of Medicine* **296**: 293–297.

7

Carotid Sinus Syncope

INTRODUCTION

Some of the structures of the head, neck and mediastinum have a unique common property. If interfered with or even when performing their normal function they may cause heart block, cardiac arrest, hypotension, syncope, seizure or sudden death. The carotid sinus is one of these structures. One common factor is the location of the structure within the afferent territory of the fifth, or more commonly, ninth, or tenth cranial nerves. The nature of the stimulus varies enormously. It may be as benign as gentle pressure on the eye (Awan, 1975), or normal swallowing. Alternatively, it may be the excruciating pain of glossopharyngeal neuralgia.

There is thus some similarity between the syncope of carotid sinus compression and syncope on swallowing in the presence of carcinoma of the oesophagus. Whatever the stimulus is, or wherever it is applied, it is more likely to cause bradycardia, asystole, or syncope if the patient is older, has arteriosclerosis, or heart disease, or is on digitalis or some other vagotonic drug.

Carotid sinus function and syncope have a long medical background. The syncope was given substantial clinical respectability by Weiss and Baker and others in the 1930s (Weiss and Baker, 1933). However, from time to time it is still reviewed with scepticism and doubt by very experienced and knowledgeable observers (Leatham, 1982).

Parry, in 1799, reporting his studies on angina pectoris, stated

> "In patients, whose hearts have been beating with undue quickness and force I have often in a few seconds retarded their motions many pulsations in a minute by strong pressure on one of the carotid arteries."

In 1866 Czermak thought that pressure on the carotid artery produced slowing of the heart by mechanical stimulation of the vagus trunk adjacent to the carotid bulb. This interpretation persisted until 1923 when Hering demonstrated slowing of the heart in animals from mechanical pressure applied directly to the bifurcation of the common carotid artery.

If the sinus is denervated these events do not occur. The fall in arterial pressure may be the result of a depressor vascular reflex alone without cardiac slowing. Following vagotomy or atropine the hypotension can occur in the absence of cardiac slowing.

Carotid sinus syncope is a somewhat ambiguous clinical condition and difficult to place in its proper perspective.

Compression of the sinus in most young people changes the pulse rate very little or not at all. In older people, particulary men and those with heart disease, it will often slow or stop the heart causing syncope. This does not mean the cause of their syncope is only a hypersensitive carotid sinus reflex.

The carotid sinus is not equally sensitive to manual compression at all times. During symptom-free periods, Walter *et al.* (1978) noted that the response to compression was normal. This fluctuating sensitivity was also noted by Peretz *et al.* (1973) and Thomas (1969).

Nevertheless, if the patient has syncope, and if his attacks are reproduced by carotid sinus compression, and a temporary pacemaker protects him from syncope on carotid compression, then permanent pacing is indicated. The site of the pathology may be in the vagus nerve or nuclei and/or the conducting system of the heart. Using carotid compression to verify and document an evanescent cardiac arrhythmia as well as the efficacy of one method of treatment appears to be an appropriate way to think about the carotid sinus reflex and to incorporate it into the clinical examination of the syncopal patient.

TYPES OF CAROTID SINUS SYNCOPE

The clinical manifestations vary. Their ease of development, intensity, and duration can be influenced by the position of the body, the state of the cerebral circulation, the heart and its conducting mechanism, and the psychological make-up and age of the individual (Thomas, 1969).

The manifestations may consist of lightheadedness only, blurring or loss of vision, generalized weakness, fullness in the head, tinnitus, tingling in the hands, dyspnoea, headache, confusion, nausea, sweating and unconsciousness.

There are two, and possibly three, kinds of carotid sinus syncope according to Weiss and co-workers (1933, 1935): cardio-inhibitory, vasopressor and central.

Cardio-inhibitory. A reflex vagal inhibition of the heart causes a fall in blood pressure as well as bradycardia. These can be prevented by atropine and epinephrine. This mechanism is the commonest and occurs in 34–78% of carotid-sinus-sensitive persons (Thomas, 1969).

Vasopressor. A fall in blood pressure, independent of changes in heart rate which is abolished by epinephrine alone is another mechanism. This is the least common form and occurs in 5–10% of patients (Thomas, 1969).

Central. Loss of consciousness occurs 3–4 sec after compression of the carotid sinus while the other forms take two or three times as long. There is no change in the heart rate or blood pressure and it is not abolished by atropine or epinephrine. This condition exists, but may be unrelated to hypersensitivity of the carotid sinus reflex. The unknown factor in this syncope is the patency of the non-compressed artery. If it was grossly stenotic or occluded and consciousness was lost on compression of the opposite carotid, this would be global cerebral ischaemia unrelated to any reflex activity of the carotid sinus.

Weiss demonstrated that stimulation of the carotid sinus in normal subjects causes no response in 30% and a fall in blood pressure of 10 mmHg or less in the remainder. However, in patients with hypertension or arteriosclerosis, carotid sinus compression caused a fall in blood pressure of 30–40 mmHg and a drop in heart rate of 8–16 beats/minute in approximately 80%. A hypersensitive carotid sinus may be found in patients with inflammatory or neoplastic disease of the neck, aneurysmal dilatation of the sinus, biliary tract disease, and following the use of certain drugs, particularly digitalis (Weiss and Baker, 1933).

Clearly the hypersensitive carotid sinus is often only one part of a wider disturbance of cardiovascular/vasomotor regulation.

Weiss and Baker (1933) studied 15 patients, 13 of whom complained of spontaneous attacks of dizziness and fainting. In four patients a sudden turn of the head induced dizziness and fainting. Pressure of graded severity on one or other carotid sinus with the patient standing produced dizziness, fainting and convulsive seizures. In the majority of cases the unconsciousness was due to marked slowing of the heart, a fall in blood pressure, or both. Three patients became syncopal on carotid pressure although there was no slowing of the heart or fall in blood pressure.

The pathology was aneurysmal dilatation of one or both carotid sinuses in six cases, a small tumour pressing on the sinus in three, and in the remaining six no abnormalities were found.

Bradycardia was present in all except three patients. Several had cardiac standstill of 2–12 sec. The slowing occurred immediately pressure was applied, but the rate became more normal even though the pressure was continued. The slowing disappeared immediately the pressure was stopped. Pressure on the eye, abdominal aorta and femoral arteries induced no slowing.

The fall in arterial blood pressure was not always related to cardiac slowing and showed wide variations. The greatest drop in blood pressure was immediately after the pressure was applied.

Stimulation of the sinus induced changes in the cardiac conducting system. These varied from patient to patient and even in the same patient at different times. The most profound changes were long periods of cardiac standstill and atrioventricular block was common. This varied from a prolonged P–R interval to complete block.

Drugs

Epinephrine was given intramuscularly and the clinical and cardiovascular effects of the reflex were abolished in all cases.

Atropine intramuscularly abolished almost entirely the reflex slowing of the pulse but not the fall in blood pressure. Sodium luminal intravenously had no effect. Novocaine block of the carotid sinus abolished the reflex slowing of the heart. Nitrites greatly accentuated the depressor reaction of the hypersensitive carotid sinus (Ferris *et al.*, 1937).

Dilatation of cerebral vessels with histamine, acetylcholine and carbon dioxide did not change the response to the sinus compression.

Ferris *et al.* (1937) studied the function of the autonomic nervous system following denervation of the hypersensitive carotid sinus. No permanent change in function occurred other than the manifestations directly associated with the hypersensitive carotid sinus syndrome.

Nathanson (1946) tested the sensitivity of the carotid sinus to compression in ambulant patients with unstated diagnosis in order to determine the incidence of what he called the 'hyperactive cardioinhibitory reflex' (HCIR). The results included only the response to compression of the *right* carotid sinus as it was usually the more effective side. A hyperactive cardio-inhibitory reflex was defined as:

1. Cardiac inhibition induced by simple pressure on the carotid sinus without massage.
2. A cardiac standstill of at least 5 sec.
3. A standstill of equal duration elicited on several tests.

Cardiac standstill as described above was induced in 115 patients, the youngest was 30 years, oldest 81 years, and the mean 59 years. It was more frequent with age and in men, the male:female ratio being 98:17. Seventy-seven patients (67%) exhibiting HCIR had no symptoms of carotid sinus syndrome. Of the remaining 38, 23 had presyncopal dizziness, or lightheadedness related to changes of position of head or body. Six patients had attacks of syncope. In each case the subjective sensations were reproducible by pressure on the carotid sinus. The cardiac inhibition was as easily elicited in the asymptomatic group as in those presenting with symptoms. Many of the group with easily induced and prolonged cardiac arrest on carotid compression could tolerate sudden movements of the head and body and tight neck-wear without symptoms.

Nathanson thought that the abnormality in the hyperactive cardio-inhibitory reflex was either in the vagus nuclei or the vagus nerve. As carotid compression may produce cardiac inhibition and a mild change in blood pressure or the reverse, the afferent side of the reflex is not at fault. There is also evidence of increased vagal activity with age, and the cardio-inhibitory response to stimulation of the carotid sinus is more frequent and intense with advanced age. The reflex is enhanced after the administration of vagus-sensitizing drugs such as digitalis and acetyl-β-methylcholine (mecholyl) (Nathanson, 1933, 1934; Weiss and Baker, 1933).

Finally, surgical denervation of the carotid sinus does not always produce a permanent cure. Although the afferent pathway has been removed, a hypersensitive vagus may be stimulated from other sites. Weiss and Ferris (1934) reported a cardiac standstill from reflex inhibition originating in a diverticulum of the oesophagus. A similar reflex may originate from the bronchi, pharynx, larynx and eye. Capps and Lewis (1907) have observed vagal reflexes induced by irritation of the pleura. The carotid sinus is but one of a number of sensory areas from which cardiac inhibition may be produced.

Nathanson concluded that: (a) a hyperactive carotid sinus reflex may be incidental and of no clinical significance; (b) the hyperactive reflex is more common with age, in males, with heart disease, and with drugs which sensitize vagus function; (c) the abnormality of the reflex is central or on the efferent side and many areas may give rise to an appropriate afferent stimulus; and (d) carotid sinus denervation may prove ineffective in reducing reflex syncopal attacks.

Draper (1950) assessed 11 unselected patients presenting with fainting or giddiness whose symptoms were reproduced by mechanical stimulation of the carotid sinus. He also found that the chief factors conditioning the response to carotid sinus pressure appeared to be age, sex, and the presence of heart disease, especially arteriosclerotic.

VASODEPRESSOR CAROTID SINUS SYNCOPE

There are few reports of vasodepressor carotid sinus syncope. Rentmeester *et al.* (1984) reported a 50-year-old man with episodes of syncope occurring after surgery and radiotherapy for a laryngeal tumour. Nine months after treatment he had two syncopal episodes with bradycardia (38/min) and hypotension (70–90/50 mmHg). Atropine relieved the bradycardia and hypotension and a temporary pacemaker was inserted. The attacks continued. He had tumour recurrence in the right carotid artery. The attacks (53 in 10 days) consisted of hypotension (blood pressure of 150–175 mmHg to 60–70 mmHg), a sharp pain in the right lateral neck radiating into the right supra-orbital region, dizziness, bradycardia (heart rate of 75–97/min to a junctional rate of about 40/min), and then syncope. Ephedrine (25 mg four times daily) and fludrocortisone (0.1 mg daily), produced substantial improvement.

Other examples of mixed bradycardia/vasodepressor carotid sinus syncope in relation to neoplasms in the neck have been reported by Patel *et al.* (1979). Pacemakers controlled the bradycardia but their three patients continued to have spells of varying degrees of hypotension.

Walter *et al.* (1978) reported 21 patients with episodes of light-headedness or syncope or both associated with a hypersensitive carotid sinus reflex. Seventeen were cardio-inhibitory, two were vasodepressor, and two were mixed. Those with more than one episode of cardio-inhibitory syncope benefited from a permanent cardiac pacemaker. The history of an event that could have stimulated the carotid sinus, i.e. neck pressure or head turning, was useful in selecting patients for pacemaker insertion.

Combined cardio-inhibitory and vasodepressor syncope may be missed unless carotid sinus stimulation is repeated after the administration of atropine.

Electrophysiological studies in 17 of these patients with cardio-inhibitory syncope suggested that sinus node dysfunction was not the cause of asystole on carotid sinus stimulation. In these 17 patients, the corrected sinus node recovery time was <525 msec in 14 and >525 msec in three patients (normal corrected time is $\ll 525$ msec). Similarly, atrioventricular conduction time was normal in 80% of their patients. Hartzler and Maloney (1977) also reported that a high proportion of their patients with cardio-inhibitory carotid sinus syncope had normal sinus node recovery time (see Gulamhusein *et al.*, 1982).

The preferred treatment for cardio-inhibitory syncope is a demand cardiac pacemaker. The results are superior to those reported from any other form of therapy.

Treatment of the vasodepressor or mixed types is more difficult. Some patients suffering vasodepressor syncope may respond to volume expansion with steroids and the mixed types may require a pacemaker plus surgical denervation of the carotid sinus.

Morley *et al.* (1982) reported 70 patients with the carotid sinus syndrome, paced and followed for four years. In an editorial commentary on this report, Leatham (1982) suggested that most, if not all, of these 70 patients had sino-atrial conduction disease. The contribution evoked from carotid sinus massage is no more or less than one might expect given the enhanced vagotonia of aging plus the underlying heart disease. The majority of Morley's patients presented with multiple syncopal episodes, the remainder with severe recurrent dizziness. A hypersensitive carotid reflex was defined as asystole or atrioventricular block for 3 sec. Carotid sinus massage was positive on the right side in 52%, on the left in 15%, and on both in 33%. Massage produced a cardio-inhibitory response in 80% of the patients while a pure vasodepressor response occurred in less than 10%.

Of the 67 patients with significant spontaneous symptoms and a hypersensitive carotid sinus reflex, 39% showed a prolonged sinus node recovery time, 16% paroxysmal atrial fibrillation and another 25% intracardiac conduction delays.

Half of all the patients had electrophysiological evidence of sino-atrial disease, either prolonged sinus node recovery time or paroxysmal atrial fibrillation precipitated by atrial pacing. This association has been noted by Mandel *et al.* (1972). None of the patients reported by Morley *et al.* had the sick sinus syndrome, although Leatham (1982) expressed serious doubts about this.

Morley believes that pacing is the treatment of choice for syncopal patients with a pure or predominantly cardio-inhibitory response to carotid sinus massage. A mixed abnormality is a therapeutic problem as ventricular pacing does not correct the vasodepressor response.

The criteria used for pacemaker implantation were hypersensitive carotid sinus reflex, reproducible symptomatic asystole longer than 3 sec, and symptomatic relief by temporary ventricular pacing during repeated massage. The effectiveness of the massage was verified by the presence of atrial asystole during temporary ventricular pacing. Ventricular demand pacing was successful in 85% of patients who were selected for this type of treatment. Twelve patients had persistent symptoms despite adequate ventricular pacing. They had significant hypotension when the 'pacemaker effect' and the vasodepressor response were combined.

Alicandri *et al.* (1978) suggested that the hypotension occurring during ventricular pacing may be related to an atrial stretch reflex activated by the high atrial pressures plus atrioventricular dissociation.

This occurs when the atria contract against closed atrioventricular valves. Eight patients were selected for atrial pacing because of improved haemodynamics demonstrated with catheter studies when the atrium was paced. All eight patients with the carotid sinus syndrome had recurrence of symptoms and symptomatic atrioventricular block from caritod sinus massage when seen in follow-up. Four of the eight who were converted to ventricular or atrioventricular pacemakers (as all eight were) continued to have symptoms after the change. Of these four, two were shown to have a combination of vasodepressor response plus pacemaker effect sufficient to explain their symptoms.

Atrioventricular sequential pacing was shown to be free of the hypotensive pacemaker effect of ventricular pacing alone, and is considered the treatment of choice for patients with carotid sinus syndrome who have both cardio-inhibitory and significant vasodepressor responses.

The patients with symptomatic vasodepressor episodes have no satisfactory treatment. In the series reported by Morley *et al.* (1982), 89% of the patients have been rendered asymptomatic with appropriate pacing systems. Forty-eight patients (68%) were asymptomatic with ventricular pacing, and fourteen with atrioventricular sequential pacing. Only four patients (6%) were likely to remain symptomatic regardless of the pacing mode due to a severe vasodepressor response.

CENTRAL CAROTID SINUS SYNCOPE

Whether carotid sinus stimulation has an effect on human cerebral activity via a purely neural mechanism is uncertain. In the cerebral or central type of carotid sinus syncope there is no change in pulse or blood pressure (Weiss and Baker, 1933).

Thomas (1972) believes it does not exist. The cerebral effects could be explained by carotid compression in subjects with an occluded contralateral carotid artery, undetected cardiovascular effects, or suggestion.

However, it has been reported that surgical manipulation in the region of the carotid sinus produced EEG slowing in two anaesthetized patients. Both had received pre-operative atropine and one was given phenylephrine hydrochloride for intra-operative hypotension. The diffuse EEG slowing was unrelated to the anaesthetic mix and was seen in the absence of bradycardia or hypotension. The carotid arteries were patent and the massage did not occlude their lumens. The EEG slowing was abolished by infiltration of lidocaine hydrochloride into the carotid sinus area (Bridgers *et al.*, 1985).

TREATMENT

Trout *et al.* (1979) treated 19 patients with the carotid sinus syndrome by carotid sinus denervation. The average age was 65.5 years and the presenting symptoms of marked dizziness or syncope were reproduced by gentle compression over the carotid bifurcation. Simultaneous ECG monitoring revealed bradycardia or transient asystole. Complete relief of symptoms or marked improvement was noted in all but one patient. Post-operative follow-up was up to 15 years. Five patients with comcomitant carotid artery stenosis had an endarterectomy at the time of denervation.

This paper adds support to the validity of carotid sinus syncope and softens Leatham's criticism of Morley's report. It has been suggested the true lesion of carotid sinus syncope is in the sino-atrial or atrioventricular conducting tissues of the heart and the carotid sinus is but an innocent precipitant capable of increasing the gain of the vagal system. If so, then denervating the sinus will produce little improvement and not for long.

Surgical procedures have also included intracranial section of the glossopharyngeal nerve (Ray *et al.*, 1948).

Vasoconstrictor and volume-expanding drugs (ephedrine and fludrocortisone) have been tried in vasodepressor or mixed carotid sinus syncope. Patel *et al.* (1979) had two patients in which ephedrine failed to control the vasodepressor manifestations. Walter *et al.* (1978) reported one patient who was symptom-free while taking fludrocortisone at 0.1 mg daily.

In the patient of Rentmeester *et al.* (1984) the combined therapy was helpful but did not completely eliminate the symptoms. The attacks were less intense and shorter.

The principal features of carotid sinus syncope are summarized in Table 7.1.

Table 7.1 Synopsis of carotid sinus syncope

- Compression of the carotid sinus can evoke asystole, atrioventricular block and syncope. Compression of the right sinus is more often effective than compression of the left
- Compression of the carotid sinus is more likely to do this in the elderly, in men more than women, and in patients with cardiac conduction abnormalities
- Carotid sinus syncope may be cardio-inhibitory, vasodepressor, or mixed. 'Central' carotid sinus syncope probably does not exist
- Carotid sinus syncope is treated with carotid sinus denervation, cardiac pacing or both. Vasodepressor syncope does not respond to pacing and is helped by fludrocortisone, ephedrine and sinus denervation

REFERENCES

Alicandri C, Fouad FM, Tarazi RC, Castle L and Morant V (1978) Three cases of hypotension and syncope with ventricular pacing. Possible role of atrial reflexes. *American Journal of Cardiology* **42**: 137–142.

Awan KJ (1975) Syncope during the removal of corneal foreign body. *Virginia Medical Monthly* **102**(5): 387–389.

Bridgers SL, Spencer SS, Spencer DD and Sasaki CT (1985) A cerebral effect of carotid sinus stimulation. Observation during intraoperative electroencephalographic monitoring. *Archives of Neurology* **42**: 574–577.

Capps JA and Lewis DD (1907) Observations upon certain blood pressure lowering reflexes that arise from irritation of the inflamed pleura. *Transactions of the Association of America Physicians* **22**: 635.

Czermak J (1866) as quoted in Weiss and Baker (1933) *Medicine* **12**: 297–354.

Draper AJ (1950) The cardio-inhibitory carotid sinus syndrome. *Annals of Internal Medicine* **32**: 700–716.

Ferris EB, Capps RB and Weiss S (1937) Relation of the carotid sinus to the autonomic nervous system and the neuroses. *Archives of Neurology and Psychiatry* **37**: 365–384.

Gulamhusein S, Naccarelli GV, Ko T, Prystowsky EN, Barnett HJM, Heger JJ and Klein GJ (1982) Value and limitations of clinical electrophysiologic study in assessment of patients with unexplained syncope. *The American Journal of Medicine* **73**: 700–705.

Hartzler CO and Maloney JE (1977) Cardio-inhibitory carotid sinus hypersensitivity. *Archives of Internal Medicine* **137**: 727–731.

Hering HE (1923) as quoted in Weiss and Baker (1933) *Medicine* **12**: 297–354.

Leatham A (1982) Carotid sinus syncope. *British Heart Journal* **47**: 409–410.

Mandel WJ, Hayakawa H, Allen HN, Danzig R and Kermaier AI (1972) Assessment of sinus node function in patients with sick sinus syndrome. *Circulation* **46**: 761–769.

Morley CA, Perrins EJ, Grant P, Chan SL, McBrien DJ and Sutton R (1982) Carotid sinus syncope treated by pacing. Analysis of persistent symptoms and role of atrioventricular sequential pacing. *British Heart Journal* **47**: 411–418.

Nathanson MH (1933) Effect of drugs on cardiac standstill induced by pressure on the carotid sinus. *Archives of Internal Medicine* **51**: 387.

Nathanson MH (1934) Further observations on the effect of drugs on induced cardiac standstill. *Archives of Internal Medicine* **54**: 111.

Nathanson MH (1946) Hyperactive cardio-inhibitory carotid sinus reflex. *Archives of Internal Medicine* **77**: 491–503.

Parry CH (1799) as quoted in Weiss and Baker (1933) *Medicine* **12**: 297–354.

Patel AK, Yap VU, Fields J and Thompson JH (1979) Carotid sinus syncope induced by malignant tumours in the neck. *Archives of Internal Medicine* **139**: 1281–1284.

Peretz DI, Gereinan AN and Miyagishima RT (1973) Permanent demand pacing for hypersensitive carotid sinus syncope. *Journal of the Canadian Medical Association* **108**: 1131–1134.

Ray BS and Stewart HJ (1948) Role of the glossopharyngeal nerve in the carotid sinus reflex in man; relief of carotid sinus syndrome by intracranial section of the glossopharyngeal nerve. *Surgery* **23**: 411–424.

Reentmeester T, Van Zile J, Van Hal M and Levene D (1984) Vasodepressor carotid sinus syncope. *British Medical Journal* **289**: 790.

Thomas JE (1969) Hyperactive carotid sinus reflex and carotid sinus syncope. *Mayo Clinic Proceedings* **44**: 127–139.

Thomas JE (1972) Disease of the carotid sinus—syncope. In: *Handbook of Clinical Neurology*, Vol 11 (eds. PH Vinken and GW Bruyn) pp. 532–551. New York: Elsevier North-Holland Inc.

Trout HH, Brown LL and Thompson JE (1979) Carotid sinus syndrome: treatment by carotid sinus denervation. *Annals of Surgery* **189**: 575–580.

Walter PF, Crawley IS and Dornay ER (1978) Carotid sinus hypersensitivity and syncope. *American Journal of Cardiology* **42**: 396–403.

Weiss S and Baker JP (1933) The carotid sinus reflex in health and disease. Its role in the causation of fainting and convulsion. *Medicine* **12**: 297–354.

Weiss S and Ferris EB (1934) Adams–Stokes syndrome with transient complete heart block of vasovagal reflex origin. *Archives of Internal Medicine* **54**: 931.

Weiss S, Wilkins RW and Haynes FW (1937) The nature of circulatory collapse induced by sodium nitrite. *Journal of Clinical Investigation* **16**: 73–84.

8

Syncope in the Young

JERVELL–LANGE-NIELSON AND ROMANO–WARD SYNDROMES

Jervell–Lange-Nielson Syndrome (Surdo-cardiac Syndrome)

In 1957 Jervell and Lange-Nielsen described four deaf siblings with heart disease. These children, between the ages of three and five, had episodes of syncope often provoked by exercise or fear. Three of the children died suddenly at ages four, five and nine years. One was still alive at age 15. ECGs from three of them revealed a marked prolongation of the Q–T interval. In one, the prolongation was even greater after exercise and quinidine, and a shortening was seen after atropine and digitalis. Mechanical systole, evaluated by phonocardiogram, was not correspondingly lengthened. None of the known causes of Q–T interval prolongation was demonstrated. T-wave changes were also seen after effort and quinidine. An autopsy of one case revealed no abnormality of the heart.

In 1958, Levine and Woodworth described an eight-year-old boy with the same disease. He had attacks of fainting from age three. The attacks were provoked by fear or fatigue. He also had a long Q–T interval, and large and often bifurcated T-waves. Clinical examination of the heart and electrolytes were normal. He died suddenly at 13 years and the heart was normal at post-mortem examination. Fraser *et al.* (1964) described nine cases of this syndrome which they named the cardio-auditory syndrome. Three of their patients died suddenly at ages $3\frac{1}{2}$, $3\frac{1}{2}$ and 14 years.

Romano–Ward Syndrome

Romano, Gemme and Pongiglione (1963) described a three-month-old child with syncopal attacks since the age of two months. The child had normal hearing and there was no familial deafness. An ECG showed ventricular fibrillation during an attack and a marked prolongation of the Q–T interval and broad diphasic T-waves between attacks. Two of this patient's brothers with identical symptoms had died at the ages of 44 days and four months, respectively.

Ward (1964) described the same clinical situation in a brother and sister. They had had syncopal attacks from the ages of 16 and 15 months, both had normal hearing and the boy died during an attack. Autopsy revealed a normal heart. Resting ECGs of both children showed extreme prolongation of the Q–T interval and during an attack, ventricular fibrillation. The mother's ECG had a prolonged Q–T interval although she was symptom-free. There was a history of sudden death in her family.

The only differences in these conditions are that the Jervell–Lange-Nielsen syndrome is associated with deafness while the Romano–Ward syndrome is not, and in the latter disease syncope occurs as early as six weeks of age.

The Attacks

There are three kind of attack:

1. Without loss of consciousness
2. With loss of consciousness and recovery
3. Those terminating fatally

Attacks without loss of consciousness have been described by Jervell and Lange-Nielsen (1957), Levine and Woodworth (1958) and Fraser *et al.* (1964). The child will stop moving, lie down or sit down and refuse to go further, grasp the chest or abdomen, and moan or cry. The pulse is normal and the attack ends within minutes. They are provoked by exertion and mental stress and the resemblance to angina is obvious. A similar episode was described in one of the patients subsequently reported by Jervell *et al.* in 1966.

Attacks with loss of consciousness or death have only been explained when an ECG was being done during an attack. They are probably due to ventricular fibrillation.

In the Romano–Ward syndrome symptoms occur as early as 2, 16, and 17 months of age. Children with the surdo-cardiac syndrome usually have their first attack later, the majority between the ages of three and seven years.

The Jervell and Lange-Nielsen syndrome may understandably be misdiagnosed as 'atypical epilepsy' (Ratshin *et al.*, 1971). Their patient was not helped by right- and left-stellate ganglion blockade, intravenous atropine, calcium gluconate or digoxin. Ventricular pacing and intravenous phenobarbitone suppressed ventricular tachyarrhythmias while sodium diphenylhydantoin produced a shortened Q–T interval and controlled the ectopic rhythms. The Romano–Ward syndrome also may be confused with epilepsy (Daly, 1981).

Sundaram *et al.* (1986) think there may be some patients in an epileptic population who are actually suffering from one of the long Q–T syndromes. Schott *et al.* (1977) have estimated that various cardiac arrhythmias from different causes can contribute to seizures in 20% of the patients diagnosed as 'idiopathic' epilepsy. They emphasized the importance of 24-h ECG monitoring to detect arrhythmias.

Although it is predominantly a disease of childhood, Furlanello *et al.* (1972) described a case of Jervell–Lange-Nielsen syndrome in a 61-year-old man whose first attack of syncope occurred at the age of 59 years. The syncope was due to ventricular fibrillation and his hearing had been impaired from an early age. His family had Q–T lengthening, syncopal episodes, pigmented naevi of the skin, and/or hearing loss, and/or a history of sudden death.

Electrocardiography

The ECG finding are remarkably consistent from one case to another and typically show a marked prolongation of the Q–T interval. The QRS complexes are normal and the prolongation, therefore, is entirely related to the ST interval and T-wave. The T-waves show many variations, being negative, bifurcated, diphasic or broad and huge. They are more abnormal after exercise and more normal after digitalis. Exercise and quinidine prolong the Q–T interval; atropine and digitalis shorten it. In some caes it has been possible to prolong the Q–T interval after exercise without a change in heart rate. After digoxin the Q–T interval decreased to just below the upper limits of normal. In addition, mechanical systole was of normal duration in contrast to electrical systole.

Pathology

Up to the report of Jervell *et al.* (1966), autopsies on five patients had demonstrated no abnormalities. James (1967) subsequently reported vascular changes in the media of the sinus nodal artery within the node and also focal fibrosis and fatty infiltration plus haemorrhage at the junction of the node with the right atrium.

Moothart *et al.* (1976) reported the cardiac electron microscopic findings of a 15-year-old boy from a family with the prolonged Q–T interval syndrome. He was the third child in the family to die suddenly on effort. Histological examination of the conduction tissues and their blood supply including the sino-atrial node, atrioventricular node, His bundle and bundle branches were normal. Myofibrils were shortened and there were abnormalities in the mitochondria which had not been reported previously.

Friedman *et al.* (1966, 1968) studied the pathology of the ear in the surdocardiac syndrome of Jervell and Lange-Nielsen. The histopathological features of two pairs of temporal bones from children who died as a result of the condition were described. A striking abnormality was the presence of PAS-positive hyalin nodules throughout both cochlear and vestibular portions of the membranous labyrinth in, or adjacent to, the terminal vessels of the vascular stria, which was atrophic. The organ of Corti was absent or degenerated and there was degeneration of the macula. The seventh and eighth cranial nerves were normal.

The report of Phillips and Ichinose (1970) is one of the few with pathological observations from a member of a family with the Romano–Ward syndrome. This patient, who died suddenly, had diffuse and extensive fibrosis of the conducting system of the heart along with abnormal changes in the sinus arterial vessels in this area. The importance of these lesions in the pathogenesis of the syndrome is not entirely clear.

According to James (1967) similar clinical manifestations have been seen in some strains of Dalmatian dogs. They have deafness, colour abnormalities of the coat and sudden death. Electrocardiograms have shown a uniform lengthening of the Q–T interval and death due to ventricular fibrillation.

Therapy

Exercise, fright and anger aggravate the condition and digitalis may be helpful. The use of propranolol in one of the patients reported by Olley and Fowler (1970) reduced the number of attacks from three or four major unconscious episodes per week to approximately one attack every 6 months. Artificial pacemaking in another patient provoked ventricular fibrillation. Schwartz *et al.* (1975) presented therapeutic data from the literature as well as from their own patients. There were 220 patients up to the date of their publication. They believed that β-adrenergic blocking agents were the treatment of choice and effective in reducing mortality. They further stated that if the syncopal attacks were not eliminated by this therapy then ablation of the left stellate ganglion along with the first thoracic ganglion was rational and specific therapy.

The patient of Landslet and Sorland (1975) with the Jervell and Lange-Nielsen syndrome who was treated for three years with a β-adrenergic blocking agent remained free of syncopal attacks for this time. Her Q–T interval remained prolonged. She had only a single syncopal attack prior to treatment. Her brother had the same syndrome with repeated attacks of syncope with and without convulsions and died suddenly. An ECG was never taken. Both children had severe iron-deficiency anaemia.

Inheritance and Other Observations on Treatment

The inheritance of the Romano–Ward syndrome has been investigated in 16 related persons by Itoh *et al.* (1982). All 10 who developed the syndrome had the same HLA haplotype (A9-Bw54) and the six who did not have the syndrome had not inherited this haplotype. The syndrome is inherited through an autosomal dominant pattern and they suggested the possibility that it is brought about by an HLA antigen gene on chromosome number 6 and other genes strongly linked to it.

Fay *et al.* (1971) surveyed 1126 deaf children in three schools for the deaf. They found one case of the surdocardiac syndrome among the 1126 children, a child formerly reported by Olley and Fowler (1970).

They discovered four other children with a history of syncope and a normal Q–T interval both at rest and after exercise. The authors thought these children represented a variant of the syndrome. In addition, they found five other children with prolonged Q–T interval but no syncope.

Mathews *et al.* (1972) reported a family with the cardio-auditory syndrome. They showed that members may have a prolonged Q–T interval and syncope with and without mild, congenital high-frequency deafness. They believed the auditory and cardiac defects were inherited separately and through an autosomal dominant mechanism in their particular family. The propositus had a prolonged Q–T interval, recurrent ventricular arrhythmias and no deafness. Intravenous diphenylhydantoin shortened the Q–T interval and intravenous phenylephrine induced ventricular fibrillation. Pathological examination of the heart in a sibling of the propositus showed areas of fibrosis in the conducting system. This patient had had his first and only unconscious episode causing his death in an automobile accident. There was no prior history of syncope, his hearing was normal, and his Q–T interval had been at the upper limits of normal (0.427).

Csandady and Kiss (1973) reported an example of the Romano–Ward syndrome. Three family members had prolonged Q–T intervals and one was resuscitated repeatedly from unconscious episodes due to ventricular fibrillation. The attacks had begun immediately after delivery and occurred at subsequent premenstrual periods. Propranolol in small doses prevented the attacks and the patient remained free of syncopal episodes despite the unchanged prolonged Q–T interval.

Hanazono *et al.* (1973) reported two unrelated females, age 21 and 17, with the Romano–Ward syndrome. Both had autosomal dominant inheritance, one heterozygous, the other homozygous, but were otherwise identical. These authors suggested that propranolol, diphenylhydantoin and phenobarbital were effective in the prevention of arrhythmias.

The disease had also been reported by Van Der Straaten and Bruins (1973) and affected individuals in their family followed an autosomal dominant pattern. In 23 family members, nine were found to have the anomaly, and of these, two at least had syncope in childhood.

Kernohan and Froggatt's (1974) patient was a 10-year-old boy with a prolonged Q–T interval, syncope, normal hearing and atrioventricular dissociation. He also had the minor attacks described in this syndrome. There were episodes with pallor, epigastric discomfort, nausea, headache but not unconsciousness. In the recovery phase there was pronounced flushing of the face and listlessness. His ECG showed atrioventricular dissociation with intermittent ventricular capture and a variable prolongation of the Q–T interval. Ventricular and atrial rates were 52 and 51/min respectively.

Isoprenaline hydrochloride increased the Q–T prolongation, while parenteral atropine produced sinus rhythm at 80 to 90 beats/min and decreased the Q–T prolongation. Parenteral diphenylhydantoin was less effective and the patient was treated with oral atropine with persistence of the minor episodes as well as the syncopal attacks.

Furberg and Hornell (1975) reported two sisters, both of whom had Q–T prolongation. One had syncope leading to epileptic seizures. Neither was deaf. The symptomatic patient was treated with propranolol with no further syncopal attacks and her ECG became normal. The asymptomatic sister was also given propranolol and her ECG became normal.

These authors emphasized that in the presence of a prolonged Q–T interval refractory periods are longer in some portions of the myocardium than others. This favours the initiation of ventricular fibrillation through the 'R-on-T phenomenon'. Q–T prolongation may also occur in myocardial necrosis, after certain stimuli to the autonomic system, and drugs such as quinidine. Biochemical, enzymatic and anatomical mechanisms have been proposed as the underlying cause of familial Q–T prolongation. A recent theory suggested asymmetrical sympathetic stimulation of the ventricular myocardium as the cause of his syndrome. Yanowitz *et al.* (1966) demonstrated that left-stellate ganglion stimulation in dogs produced a prolonged Q–T interval. More recently, Moss and McDonald (1971) demonstrated, in a patient with Q–T prolongation, that left-stellate ganglion block produced a normal Q–T interval while a block on the right caused further prolongation. After a left-stellate ganglionectomy the Q–T interval became normal and there were no further syncopal episodes. They had been documented as due to ventricular fibrillation. Although propranolol appears to be the treatment of choice (Gale *et al.*, 1970; Garza *et al.*, 1970), it is not always effective and usually does not alter the Q–T interval. The two patients of Furberg and Hornell (1975) had normal Q–T intervals after starting propranolol.

Frank and Friedberg (1976) reported four children with syncope and prolonged Q–T intervals, one of whom was deaf. All were treated with propranolol, eliminating the syncope, while the ECGs were unchanged.

The family of Anderson and Lundkvist (1979) demonstrated the variability of the disease within a single family. They described nine brothers and sisters of whom five were deaf. Two of the siblings died without examination while ECGs of the other three showed prolonged Q–T intervals. Two of the five had not had more than a single syncope since puberty and were alive and well. The other three had frequent attacks into their adult years and died in syncopal episodes at aged 20, 27 and 37.

Increased Heart Rate and Decreased Q–T Interval

DiSegni *et al.* (1980) treated nine patients with prolonged Q–T intervals and syncope by overdrive pacing. Six of the patients were receiving quinidine sulphate for atrial fibrillation or premature beats, two were on prenylamine for angina pectoris, and the ninth was a newborn with a congenitally long Q–T interval. Prolongation of the Q–T interval may be associated with repetitive attacks of ventricular tachycardia of the 'torsade de pointes' type (see below) or of ventricular fibrillation. These authors used endocardial pacing in all nine patients. Acceleration of the heart rate resulted in immediate suppression of all arrhythmias. Pacing was continued until the condition producing the Q–T prolongation disappeared, except in the newborn in which it was permanent. Overdrive pacing shortened the absolute Q–T interval from a mean of 0.65 sec to 0.50 sec. The corrected Q–T interval remained prolonged (about 0.56 sec). The arrhythmia, therefore, was related to the duration of the actual Q–T interval and overdrive pacing inhibited it without shortening the corrected Q–T interval.

Syncope as a complication of quinidine therapy has been recognized since the drug was introduced as an anti-arrhythmic. Syncope may occur in 5% of attempted quinidine conversions of atrial flutter or fibrillation and the incidence increases with higher doses, but may not be dose-related at all. The syncope of quinidine is associated with a prolongation of the Q–T interval and ventricular arrhythmia, either fibrillation or paroxysms of tachycardia. It is characterized by 'the continuously changing configuration and electrical axes of the ventricular complexes as if they were twisting around the isoelectric line' (DiSegni *et al.*, 1980). This configuration is known as 'torsade de pointes'. These episodes may stop spontaneously or go on to fibrillation. Torsade de pointes was identified in eight of the nine patients described by DiSegni *et al.* and changed to ventricular fibrillation in five. The mechanism of the changing axis and configuration of the 'torsade' is not known. Prolongation of the Q–T interval is due to increased time for ventricular repolarization and the repolarization time may not be the same in all ventricular fibres (Rossi and Matturri, 1976). This inequality of excitability predisposes the heart to various arrhythmias. DiSegni has hypothesized that quinidine, other drugs, and some diseases prolong repolarization (and therefore the Q–T interval) but unevenly, thus leading to the temporal dispersion of recovery and arrhythmia. This would naturally be enhanced by pre-existing, myocardial pathology, i.e. ischaemia, hypertrophy and conduction disturbances.

If the above is correct, rational treatment of the prolonged Q–T syndrome would be reduction of the spread of repolarization by acceleration of the heart rate. Heart rate is inversely related to the temporal dispersion of repolarization. DiSegni *et al.* successfully used isoproterenol for this purpose in three of their patients, but then decided that the preferred and safer method of acceleration was electrical pacing at a higher rate than the intrinsic heart rate, i.e. overdrive pacing. This proved effective at rates from 90–120 beats/min and caused no haemodynamic problem, angina or undesirable side-effects. They noted that overdrive pacing shortened the Q–T interval, but the corrected Q–T interval remained prolonged and it is the duration of the absolute Q–T interval that represents the degree of temporal dispersion of repolarization.

Clearly, overdrive pacing needs further consideration in the treatment of prolonged Q–T interval syncope in cases other than those due to quinidine and other drugs.

Hartzler and Osborn (1981) performed electrophysiological studies on a seven-year-old boy with the Jervell–Lange-Nielsen syndrome. They found increased ventricular refractoriness and were unable to induce ventricular fibrillation. The electrophysiological responses were improved following left-stellate block. However, left-stellate sympathectomy was followed by spontaneous ventricular fibrillation, and an unchanged Q–T interval.

Von Bernuth *et al.* (1982) reported two groups of children with syncope with stress or exercise. One group, some of whom were deaf, had resting Q–T prolongation while the other group had normal Q–T intervals. The stress or exercise-induced syncope was due to some type of ventricular dysrhythmia, most commonly a junctional tachycardia, ventricular bigeminy or ventricular tachycardia. Three of the latter group died during syncopal episodes, and one suffered severe hypoxic brain damage during an attack. Both groups were improved by treatment with β-adenergic blocking medication.

Packer *et al.* (1984) report a 14-year-old girl with normal hearing and no family history of deafness. She had syncope after exertion and palpitations, dizziness and light-headedness when anxious. She had a prolonged Q–T interval. Left stellatectomy and continuing β-adrenergic blocking drugs did not prevent her death seven months after the operation. She died with ventricular fibrillation and was one of three late deaths among 53 patients who have undergone stellactectomy for the prolonged Q–T syndrome (Schwartz and Locati, 1985).

OTHER CAUSES OF CHILDHOOD SYNCOPE

There are reported cases of syncope or Adams–Stokes attacks in children due to ventricular fibrillation without organic disease of the heart and with a normal Q–T interval (Berg, 1960; Wennevold *et al.*, 1965). Thus, there are three childhood syndromes with syncope, Adams–Stocks attacks, and no signs of organic heart disease between attacks:

- the surdocardiac syndrome (Jervell–Lange-Nielsen)
- the same without deafness (Romano–Ward)
- syncope with multiple extrasystoles and ventricular fibrillation, without deafness and a normal Q–T interval

Paroxysmal Ventricular Fibrillation and the Short P–R Interval

McRae *et al.* (1974) described a family in which three siblings had syncopal episodes and sudden death; a fourth had syncopal episodes and proven paroxysmal ventricular fibrillation. Important characteristics of the ECG were a short P–R interval and prominent U-waves. The episodes of fibrillation were induced by stressful emotional stimuli and not by exercise. The surviving patient was successfully maintained symptom-free on propanolol for many years.

Assorted Dysrhythmias

Beder *et al.* (1985) evaluated six children with syncope of unknown aetiology. Neurological evaluation, cardiac examination, chest x-ray, and two-dimensional echocardiograms were normal in all. Abnormal findings in five patients included Mobitz Type II atrioventricular block, sinus bradycardia (three patients), and supraventricular tachycardia (one patient). Four patients had one or more abnormal findings on electrophysiological studies, including sinus node dysfunction (three patients), atrioventricular node dysfunction (three patients), and distal His-Purkinje system disease (two patients). All had normal right heart haemodynamic catheter studies. Clearly, arrhythmias are an important cause of syncope in some children with an otherwise normal heart.

Breath-holding Spell and Pain-induced Syncope

These have been known since 1616 (Culpepper). The child may be frightened, hurt or angry.

He will then cry vigorously for a few breaths and then hold his breath. He rapidly becomes cyanosed, unconscious, limp and falls. He may have a few jerks of his limbs or increased tonus of the whole body and the attack is then over.

Lombroso and Lerman (1967) assessed 92 children because of breath-holding spells The age of onset varied from the neonatal period to 42 months, with a maximum incidence between 7 and 18 months af age. All the attacks stopped spontaneously except in two, aged $7\frac{1}{2}$ and $6\frac{1}{2}$ years. They found that epilepsy and mental deficiency were unrelated to breath-holding attacks while syncope in adults was a common sequel of breath-holding in infancy. They divided the patients into two groups, cyanotic or pallid. The prognosis for both types was excellent. In the pallid group, if the attacks were frequent, atropine was found to be helpful, but the treatment in most instances was unnecessary.

Lombroso and Lerman suggested the explanation for the attacks is: (1) violent crying, with forced, lengthy expiration leads to hypocapnoeic cerebral ischaemia; (2) apnaeic hypoxaemia; and (3) an effective valsalva with increased intrathoracic pressure, reduced atrial filling, reduced cardiac output, central arterial and pulmonary compression, impaired cerebral circulation added to the other mechanisms leading to unconsciousness. This mechanism is simliar to the 'mess trick' (see Chapter 9) and some kinds of cough syncope.

Laxdal *et al.* (1969) oberved 184 children with breath-holding spells. They clearly differentiated two types of spells. The pallid spell is almost always a consequence of a sudden, unexpected, painful stimulus. The child will gasp without crying, become apnoeic, and unresponsive. The latter type of pain-induced syncope is probably unrelated to breath holding *per se,* as it is often familial and lifelong. The cyanotic, crying, apnoeic, spell almost always disappears during more mature childhood and is rarely, if ever, seen in adults.

In contrast, syncope in response to pain is almost certainly a brain-stem reflex producing unconsciousness by means of a transient dysrhythmia or asystole. A doctor (personal communication) reported that if he hurt himself severely and unexpectly (struck his thumb with a hammer) he could feel himself fading into unconsciousness *before* he felt the pain in his thumb. On recovery, the pain in the thumb was the only complaint and this diminished over the next 3–5 min suggesting he had been unconscious probably not more than 30 or 60 sec. His father had the same response to pain as did his son.

There is no evidence that this phenomenon has any relationship to breath holding and the concept of 'cyanotic' and 'pallid' breath-holding spells is spurious. The former is hypoxic, hypocapnoeic, valsalva-induced, defective cerebral perfusion; the latter is a pain-induced vasovagal reflex.

Syncope in Asthmatic Children Following Epinephrine

Speer and Tapay (1970) described four children, all asthmatics, with syncope or near-syncope following the use of epinephrine. The drug produced profound tachycardia, hypotension and cardiac dysrhythmias as well. There were no fatalities although they have occurred in this situation.

Adolescent Syncope

Risser (1985) believed the commonest faint in adolescents is vasodepressor vasovagal in response to anger, fear, anxiety or pain.

Migraine, according to Risser, is another common cause of syncope in adolescents. It is

Table 8.1 Synopsis of syncope in the young

- Familial deafness, prolonged Q–T interval, syncope and sudden death in children is a syndrome of unknown cause called the Jervell–Lange-Nielsen and surdo-cardiac syndrome
- A similar syndrome without the deafness but with syncope and sudden death in infancy is called the Romano–Ward syndrome
- The children have attacks without syncope in which they squat, grasp the chest or abdomen, moan or cry
- Overdrive pacing producing a faster heart rate may reduce the increased time of ventricular repolarization (the prolonged Q–T interval) thereby eliminating the inequality of ventricular fibre excitability and arrhythmias
- Syncope also occurs in children with multiple extrasystoles, ventricular fibrillation, no deafness and a normal Q–T interval
- Breath-holding spells are benign with a good prognosis and are due to an extended and forceful valsalva manoeuvre
- So-called 'pallid breath-holding spells' are vasovagal, pain-initiated syncope and unrelated to cyanotic true breath-holding

usually basilar with visual disturbance, ataxia, dysaesthesiae in the hands, feet, and lips, vertigo, dysarthria and tinnitus. The headache is generally occipital and subarachnoid haemorrhage must be seriously considered in the differential diagnosis.

Hyperventilation can produce unconsciousness but is a very uncommon cause.

Syncope in young people can be due to mitral-valve prolapse. The syncope or near-syncope in this disease may be caused by transient cerebral ischaemia or by dysrhythmias which are relatively frequent. The disorder is diagnosed by a mid-systolic click at the apex followed by a late systolic murmur and echocardiography is necessary to confirm the diagnosis. The heart must be listened to with the patient in different positions (Barnett *et al.*, 1980). Mitral-valve prolapse is at times associated with scoliosis, a pectus excavatum, or an abnormally straight back with loss of the normal thoracic curve.

The 'ophthalmoplegia plus' of Kearns–Sayre syndrome includes ophthalmoplegia, retinitis, short stature, neurological disorders, and a Q–T interval which is prolonged. Occasionally the prolongation is only during exercise.

Aortic stenosis and idiopathic hypertrophic subaortic stenosis with outflow obstruction can lead to syncope particularly on exercise (Chapter 5).

Pulmonary hypertension and pulmonary stenosis are also causes of syncope in the young and are described in Chapter 9. Cough syncope occurs in youngsters, particularly teenagers, and is described in Chapter 9 also.

A synopsis of syncope in the young is shown in Table 8.1.

REFERENCES

Andersson P and Lunkdvist L (1979) Q–T Syndrome—a family description. *Axta Medica Scandinavica* **206**: 73–76.

Barnett HJ, Boughner DR, Taylor DW, Cooper PE, Kostuk WJ and Nichol PM (1980) Further evidence relating mitral valve prolapse to cerebral ischemic events. *New England Journal of Medicine* **302**: 139–144.

Beder SD, Cohen, MH and Riemenschneider TA (1985) Occult arrhythmias as the etiology of unxplained syncope in children with structurally normal hearts. *American Heart Journal* **109**(2): 309–313.

Berg KH (1960) Multifocal ventricular extrasystoles with Adams–Stokes syndrome in siblings. *American Heart Journal* **60**: 965.

Csandady M and Kiss Z (1973) Heritable Q–T prolongation without congenital deafness (Romano–Ward syndrome). *Chest* **64**(3): 359–362.

Culpepper T, in Lennox WG and Lennox M (1960) *Epilepsy and Related Disorders*. pp. 389–392. Boston: Little Brown & Co.

Daly RF (1981) *Handbook of Clinical Neurology* **42**: 718–719.

DiSegni E, Klein HO, David D, Libhaber C and Kaplinsky E (1980) Overdrive pacing in quinidine syncope and other long Q–T interval syndromes. *Archives of Internal Medicine* **140**: 1036–1040.

Fay JE, Olley PM, Partington MW, Kavety VB and Ahmad G (1971) Surdo-cardiac syndrome: incidence among children in schools for the deaf. *Canadian Medical Association Journal* **105**(7): 718–720.

Frank JP and Friedberg DZ (1976) Syncope with prolonged Q–T interval. *American Journal of Diseases of Childhood* **130**(3): 320–322.

Fraser GR, Froggatt P and James TN (1964) Congenital deafness associated with electrocardiographic abnormalities, fainting attacks, and sudden deaths. *Quarterly Journal of Medicine* **33**: 361–385.

Friedmann, I, Fraser GR and Froggatt P (1966) Pathology of the ear in cardio-auditory syndrome of Jervell and Lange-Nielsen (recessive deafness with electrocardiographic abnormalities). *Journal of Laryngology* **80**(5): 451–470.

Friedmann, I, Fraser GR and Froggatt P (1968) Pathology of the ear in cardio-auditory syndrome of Jervell and Lange-Nielsen. *Journal of Laryngology* **82**: 883.

Furberg C and Hornell H (1975) Familial Q–T prolongation and risk of sudden death. *Acta Pediatrica Scandinavica* **64**: 777–782.

Furlanello F, Macca F and Dal Palu C (1972) Observations on a case of Jervell and Lange-Nielsen syndrome in an adult. *British Heart Journal* **34**: 648–652.

Gale GE, Bosman CK, Tucker RBK and Barlow JB (1970) Hereditary prolongation of the Q–T interval: study of two families. *British Heart Journal* **32**: 505.

Garza LA, Vick RL, Nora JJ and McNamara DG (1970) Heritable Q–T prolongation without deafness. *Circulation* **41**: 39.

Hanazono N, Ando Y, Ohnishi M. Oda H, Yuhara N, Nishio T, Ishida H, Takeuchi A and Kohashi K (1973) Heritable Q–T prolongation without deafness: the Romano–Ward syndrome. *Japanese Heart Journal* **14**(6): 479–493.

Hartzler GO and Osborn MJ (1981) Invasive electrophysiological studies in the Jervell and Lange-Nielsen syndrome. *British Heart Journal* **45**: 225–229.

Itoh S, Munemura S and Satoh H (1982) A study of the inheritance pattern of Romano–Ward syndrome. *Clinical Pediatrics* **21**: 20–24.

James TN (1967) Congenital defects and cardiac arryhthmias. *American Journal of Cardiology* **19**: 627–643.

Jervell A and Lange-Nielsen F (1957) Congenital deaf mutism, functional heart disease with prolongation of the Q–T interval and sudden death. *American Heart Journal* **54**: 59.

Jervell A, Thingstead R and Endsjo T-O (1966) The surdo-cardiac syndrome. *American Heart Journal* **72**(5): 582–593.

Kernohan RJ and Froggatt P (1974) Atrioventricular dissociation with prolonged Q–T interval and syncopal attacks in a 10 year old boy. *British Heart Journal* **36**: 516–519.

Langslet A and Sorland SJ (1975) Surdo-cardiac syndrome of Jervell and Lange-Nielsen with prolonged Q–T interval present at birth and severe anaemia and syncopal attacks in childhood. *British Heart Journal* **37**: 830–832.

Laxdal T, Gomez MR and Reiher J (1969) Cyanotic and pallid syncopal attacks in children (breath holding spells). *Develop Med Child Neurol* **11**: 755–763.

Levine SA and Woodworth CR (1958) Congenital deaf mutism, prolonged Q–T interval, syncopal attacks, and sudden death. *New England Journal of Medicine* **259**: 412.

Lombroso CT and Lerman T (1967) Breath holding spells (cyanotic and pallid infantile syncope). *Pediatrics* **39**(4): 563–581.

Mathews EC, Blount AW and Townsend JI (1972) Q–T prolongation and ventricular arrhythmias, with and without deafness, in the same family. *American Journal of Cardiology* **29**(5): 720–721.

McRae JR, Wagner GS, Rogers MC and Canent RV (1974) Paroxysmal familial ventricular fibrillation. *Journal of Pediatrics* **84**(4): 515–518.

Moothart RW, Pryor R, Hawley RL, Clifford NJ and Blount SG (1976) The heritable syndrome of prolonged Q–T interval syncope and sudden death. *Chest* **70**(2): 203–266.

Moss AJ and McDonald J (1971) Unilateral cervico-thoracic sympathetic ganglionectomy for the treatment of long Q–T interval syndrome. *New England Journal of Medicine* **285**: 903.

Olley PM and Fowler RS (1970) The surdo-cardiac syndrome: haemodynamic and therapeutic observations. *British Heart Journal* **32**: 467–471.

Packer DL, Coltorti F, Smith MS, Bardy GH, Benson DW, Edwards SB and German LD (1984) Sudden death after left stellectomy in the long Q–T syndrome. *American Journal of Cardiology* **54**(10): 1365–1366.

Phillips J and Ichinose H (1970) Clinical and pathological studies in the hereditary syndrome of a long Q–T interval, syncopal spells, and sudden death. *Chest* **58**(3): 236–243.

Ratshin RA, Hunt D, Russell RO and Rackley CE (1971) Q–T interval prolongation, paroxysmal ventricular arrhythmias, and convulsive syncope. *Annals of Internal Medicine* **75**(6): 919–924.

Risser WL (1985) Syncope in adolescents. *American Family Physicians* **32**(5): 117–123.

Romano C, Gemme G and Pongiglione R (1963) Aritmie cardiache rare dell 'eta' pediatrica. *La Clinica Pediatrica* **45**: 656.

Rossi L and Matturri L (1976) Histopathologic findings in two cases of torsades de pointes with conduction disturbances. *British Heart Journal* **38**: 1312–1318.

Schott GD, McLeod AA and Jewitt DE (1977) Cardiac arrhythmias that masquerade as epilepsy. *British Medical Journal* **1**: 1454–1457.

Schwartz PJ and Locati E (1985) The idiopathic long Q–T syndrome. Pathogenetic mechanisms and therapy. *European Heart Journal* **6** (**supplement D**): 103–114.

Schwartz PJ, Periti M and Malliani A (1975) The long Q–T syndrome. *American Heart Journal* **89**(3): 378–390.

Speer F and Tapay NJ (1970) Syncope in children following epinephrine. *Annals of Allergy* **28**(2): 50–54.

Sundaram MBM, McMeekin JD and Gulamhusein S (1986) Cardiac tachyarrhythmias in hereditary long Q–T syndromes presenting as a seizure disorder. *Canadian Journal of Neurological Sciences* **13**(3): 262–263.

Van der Straaten PJC and Bruins CLD (1973) A family with heritable electrocardiographic Q–T prolongation. *Journal of Medical Genetics* **10**: 158–160.

Von Bernuth G, Bernsaw U, Gutheil H, Hoffmann W. Huschke U, Jungst BK, Kallfelz HS, Lang D, Sandhage K, Schmaltz AA, Schmidt-Redemann B, Weber H and Weiner C (1982) Tachyarrhythmic syncopes in children with structurally normal hearts with and without Q–T prolongation in the electrocardiogram. *European Journal of Pediatrics* **138**: 206–210.

Ward OC (1964) A new familial cardiac syndrome in children. *Journal of the Irish Medical Association* **54**: 103.

Wennevold A, Melchior JC and Sandoe E (1965) Adams–Strokes syndrome in children without organic heart disease. *Acta Medica Scandinavica* **177**: 557.

Yanowitz F, Preston JB and Abildskov JA (1966) Functional distribution of right and left stellate innervation to the ventricles: production of neurogenic electrocardiographic changes by unilateral alteration of sympathetic tone. *Circulation Research* **18**: 416.

9

Pulmonary Disease, Coughing and Syncope

INCREASED INTRATHORACIC PRESSURE

About 75% of the total blood volume is in the venous side of the circulation and its flow towards the heart is partially dependent on the small pressure gradient between the venous end of the capillaries and the right atrium. When standing, gravity adds venous pooling and retards venous return accounting for the 30% decrease in cardiac output in the upright position.

A sudden increase in intrathoracic pressure can eliminate this small but critical pressure gradient and reduce venous return and cardiac output, which in turn causes syncope. Examples are attempted expiration against a closed glottis (the valsalva manoeuvre, straining at the toilet, lifting a heavy object and deliberate breath-holding. In the syncope of prolonged coughing an additional element is thought to be the concussive effect of each cough through the veins against the cerebrospinal fluid. This results in compression and inhibition of the filling of the intracranial vascular bed.

PULMONARY HYPERTENSION

Pulmonary hypertension, either primary or secondary, may be complicated by syncopal episodes. The syncope usually occurs on effort. It also occurs with right ventricular outflow obstruction such as congenital pulmonary stenosis and the tetralogy of Fallot.

The mechanism is the failure of the right ventricle to increase its output on demand. If there is no right-to-left shunt, cor pulmonale develops plus inadequate left ventricle output and hypotension. (What the right ventricle can do determines what the left ventricle may do.) When a shunt is present, its capacity increases with further systemic arterial hypoxia. The syncope may be due directly to cerebral ischaemia or a vasodepressor reflex may be set off by stimulation of thoracic or cardio/aortic baroreceptors. Sudden death occurs frequently.

Effort syncope may be an early and the only manifestation of primary pulmonary hypertension. It may precede the manifestations of right-ventricle hypertrophy and dilatation of the pulmonary artery. Effort syncope was the presenting symptom in three cases of primary pulmonary hypertension reported by Dressler (1952) and in six other cases in the literature. They all had common features: (a) syncope precipitated by effort, (b) dilatation of the pulmonary artery, and (c) right-ventricular hypertrophy with no obvious cause. Physiological studies revealed marked pulmonary hypertension. Autopsy examination revealed pulmonary arteriosclerosis in five patients, but in two it was mild and insufficient to explain the right-ventricular hypertrophy.

In all cases the syncope occurred on effort and as the disease advanced less effort was required to produce it. The premonitory symptoms were the same as in syncope from other causes, i.e. light-headedness, epigastric distress, choking and chest tightness. The syncopal attacks lasted from a few seconds to minutes and in one case 25 min. Cyanosis and muscular rigidity were often present and some patients were incontinent. The episodes were often followed by nausea, vomiting, cramps and diarrhoea. The frequency of syncopal attacks varied from two to a dozen or were innumerable.

Mechanisms

Increased pressure in the pulmonary vasculature can cause bradycardia and systemic hypotension (Harrison *et al.*, 1932; Parin, 1947). The increased pressure in the pulmonary conus will cause cardiac slowing, and the elevated pulmonary venous pressure initiates the systemic hypotension. These reflex mechanisms contribute to the syncope of positive pressure breathing, pulmonary oedema, congestive heart failure, coughing, pulmonary hypertension and pulmonary embolus.

However, the mechanism of syncope in pulmonary hypertension is not clear. It is not always related to cyanosis, arterial oxygen level or cerebral hypoxia.

Syncope has been observed during exercise testing in patients with pulmonary hypertension. Neither pulse nor heart sounds were found during the unconscious state. On recovery, the heart remained slow and irregular for some time suggesting a component of vagal over-activity. Raising the pressure in the pulmonary artery of experimental animals will decrease systemic arterial pressure and pulse rate (Daly *et al.*, 1937). This reflex is abolished by cutting the pulmonary branches of the vagus nerve.

HYPERVENTILATION SYNCOPE

Although hyperventilation is a common symptom, it rarely causes unconsciousness. One hundred and sixty-five volunteers were hyperventilated until they had muscle incoordination, but none fainted (Wayne, 1958). However, patients who may be more emotionally involved with the process and hyperventilate for fun or gain are more likely to faint. Possible mechanisms include an increase in peripheral blood flow with splanchnic and muscle vasodilatation with resulting hypotension (Brown, 1953). In addition, ECG changes occur which have been interpreted as ischaemic (Bloom, 1946). Relatively mild hyperventilation can reduce cerebral blood flow by as much as 35% (Kety and Schmidt, 1946; Patterson *et al.*, 1951). In addition, the increased affinity of haemoglobin for oxygen in the presence of hypocapnoea contributes to the cerebral hypoxia. Any of these abnormalities may contribute to loss of consciousness in a susceptible hyperventilating person.

COUGH SYNCOPE

Cough syncope was first described by Heberden in 1802 and again by Charcot in 1876. More than 300 cases have since been reported. In its common form it is usually a complaint of middle-aged men who suffer from chronic bronchitis, emphysema, are overweight and heavy smokers.

The fainting episode is always associated with a paroxysm of vigorous coughing. There is light-headedness followed by unconsciousness and quick recovery. There is rarely incontinence or convulsive activity and there is no post-ictal drowsiness or confusion.

Hard coughing elevates intrathoracic pressure, impedes venous return and decreases cardiac output (Sharpey-Schafer, 1953). Additionally, the high intrathoracic pressure during cough is transmitted to the subarachnoid space, which further reduces cerebral blood flow. Kerr and Eich (1966) have suggested that the rapid rise in intracranial pressure might have a 'concussion'-like effect in contributing to the loss of consciousness.

Pedersen *et al.* (1966) assessed five patients with typical cough syncope. Haemodynamic investigations including simultaneous measurements of pressure in the pulmonary and systemic circulations were carried out. Intrathoracic pressure was measured via a catheter in the oesophagus. Pressures were measured during graded valsalva manoeuvre and paroxysms of coughing brought on by smoking. Three of the patients fainted while the pressures were being measured, while two could not be induced to faint at all.

The valsalva manoeuvre and coughing produced similar abnormalities. The findings in the five patients subjected either to the valsalva manoeuvre or coughing were as follows:
The pressure within the intrathoracic portion of the venous circulation rose abruptly and was exactly parallel with the intrathoracic pressure. The pressure within the peripheral venous system rose at a slower rate, presumably because this system, with its larger volume of blood and partially filled vessels, required a greater increase of volume before increasing the pressure. For a brief period the peripheral venous pressure was lower than the pressure in the intrathoracic veins. The venous circulation was impeded at the entrance to the thorax. The stroke volume of the ventricles decreased rapidly (Booth *et al.*, 1962), first the right and then the left, causing a fall in systemic arterial pressure. As the cough or valsalva continued the pressure in the peripheral veins increased and the pressure gradient from artery to vein was diminished, resulting in impaired peripheral blood flow.

There was no evidence of a vagal component to the syncope. The length and strength of the coughing are both greater in those who faint compared to those who do not. Most normal people cannot cough long enough or hard enough to produce the required increase in intrathoracic pressure (McIntosh *et al.*, 1956; Pederson *et al.*, 1966).

Skolnick and Dines (1969) reported the details of 18 patients with cough syncope seen in the Mayo Clinic over a 17-year period. They estimated that a single cough would increase intrathoracic pressure 20–30 mmHg and a more vigorous cough could increase it to 100 mmHg. The cough associated with syncope will generally produce a pressure of 100–300 mmHg.

Emphysematous patients have several predisposing factors to cough syncope. Their alveolar pressure is greater than normal and hence an even higher pressure may develop during coughing. They have greater variations of intrapleural pressure and increased rigidity of peripheral alveoli, preventing full transmission of pressure from within the tracheobronchial tree to the pleural spaces. They also have a lower intra-alveolar oxygen content.

Corson (1970) thought that coughing in normal subjects and patients with emphysema raised intrathoracic pressure from 50 to 150 mmHg, while coughing in patients with cough syncope produced pressures from 200 to 300 mmHg.

Cough, Sneeze Syncope, Atlanto-occipital Junction Abnormalities, Arnold-Chiari Malformation, Syringobulbia, Syringomyelia and Hydrocephalus

Larson *et al.* (1974) reported two patients with cough syncope and herniated cerebellar tonsils apparently of congenital origin. Neither had hydrocephalus and both were cured by sub-occipital craniectomy and upper cervical laminectomy.

> *Case 1.* Examining the first patient during coughing revealed that the cerebrospinal fluid pressure rose and then fell to below the resting level, the transmitted pulse pressure waves disappeared, hypotension, bradycardia, and occipital headache developed, and somatosensory evoked potential amplitudes were markedly reduced. The patient's complaints were headache induced by coughing associated with paraesthesiae in the hands, cold sweat, dizziness, ataxia, light-headedness and ultimately syncope. Within 30 sec after the onset of coughing, the blood pressure which had been 120/90 mmHg fell to 80/60 mmHg and pulse rate to 60/min (it had been 90/min). One minute after coughing, blood pressure and pulse rate returned to resting values. Somatosensory-evoked potential amplitudes returned to normal values and the headache disappeared 2 min after the end of coughing. A cervical laminectomy and occipital craniectomy were done. The cerebellar tonsils were found 1.5 cm below the rim of the foramen magnum. There were no further episodes of cough syncope or syncope in the next two years.
>
> *Case 2.* The second patient, a man of 48 years, sneezed and lost consciousness. On another occasion he bent over to pick up a shovel and lost consciousness. Both episodes had syncopal characteristics and he also had a history of cough syncope. His cerebellar tonsils were found to be herniated into the cervical canal. Lumbar puncture was done and the patient could not cough sufficiently to raise the CSF pressure. The Chiari Type I malformation was relieved by occipital craniectomy and laminectomy and he had no further syncope.

The findings in these patients suggest that prior to surgery, coughing further impacted the tonsils into the foramen magnum occluding the subarachnoid space. The compression of the medulla contributed to the decrease in blood pressure and subsequent faintness. The somatosensory evoked potential recordings support the hypothesis of intermittent medullary compression.

Corbett *et al.* (1976) reported the following case:

> *Case Study.* A 29-year-old man had dizziness and unconsciousness after sneezing, for the previous 15 years. On sneezing he had a 'crick' in his neck, dizziness, vertigo, and then nausea which would persist for up to 15 min. He might have a period of unconsciousness for 3 or 4 sec. Not all sneezes were effective. There was a history of a positive Lhermitte's phenomenon. He noted that straining during bowel movements or isometric exercises produced an identical sequence of events. Investigation and surgery revealed an Arnold–Chiari Type I malformation with herniation of the cerebellar tonsils to C3. Sub-occipital craniectomy and decompression laminectomy alleviated all symptoms.

These authors point out that a sudden increase in intrathoracic or intra-abdominal pressure, as in the valsalva manoeuvre, causes an instantaneous increase in CSF pressure equal to the intrathoracic pressure as well as a brief increase in blood pressure. Blood pressure and pulse pressure then drop rapidly and slowly rise with the pulse rate until the glottis opens. The decreased cardiac filling pressure and the drop in output and atrial pressure produce cerebral ischaemia and at times unconsciousness.

Williams (1980) has explained syncope (and headache) from coughing, sneezing, or effort, in chronic hind-brain herniation on the differential pressures of CSF above and below the foramen magnum. The timing of the increased pressure in the two compartments is also different in chronic hind-brain hernia.

In normal subjects, raising abdominal and thoracic pressure distends Batson's plexus of veins, compresses the theca and CSF flows from the spinal to the cranial compartment. With an obstructed foramen magnum, intracranial pressure temporarily exceeds spinal pressure. The hind-brain hernia impacts and the medulla is possibly temporarily ischaemic and/or unable to carry out its baroreceptor functions.

Hampton *et al.* (1982) reported three patients with syringomyelia presenting with syncope. All had evidence of hind-brain herniation into the cervical canal and all were improved following craniovertebral decompression. The differential pressure response between lumbar and ventricular spinal fluid pressures on forced expiration was also returned to normal by the surgical procedure.

Dobkin (1978) described a 42-year-old man with syncopal episodes induced by modest exertion. Pedalling a stationary bicycle for 30 sec, bilateral jugular vein compression for 15–30 sec, or a valsalva manoeuvre for 10–15 sec at an expiratory pressure of 30 mmHg, caused syncope. Arterial blood pressure, gases and heart rate were unchanged prior to, during, and after the loss of consciousness except during phase II of the valsalva manoeuvre when the blood pressure dropped by the normal average value of 10–15% while heart rate increased 20–25%.

Investigations revealed displacement of the fourth ventricle and cerebellar tonsils below the foramen magnum. Sub-occipital craniectomy and upper cervical laminectomy confirmed the diagnosis and relieved the symptoms.

Cough Syncope and Idiopathic Hypertrophic Subaortic Stenosis (IHSS)

White *et al.* (1975) reported a case of idiopathic hypertrophic sub-aortic stenosis presenting as cough syncope. This is a unique patient with enough reduction in systemic blood pressure during and after coughing to render him unconscious. White and his colleagues performed a careful and informative study. It provides physiological data on some of the transient abnormalities on hard and sustained coughing. Syncope (unrelated to coughing) is a common symptom in this disease and the cause is not well understood.

Case study. The patient, a 45-year-old man, complained of progressive dyspnoea and episodes of dizziness following coughing, once or twice a month occasionally leading to unconsciousness. Blood pressure was 170/95 and pulse 80 per minute. A grade 3/6 systolic ejection murmur was heard which increased during the valsalva manoeuvre, on standing, with amyl nitrate inhalation, and decreased with isometric hand grip.

Left-ventricle hypertrophy and left-atrial enlargement were identified. Respiratory functions were normal. Coughing on request for 5 sec produced intrathoracic pressure of 250 mmHg. The pressure remained 5–10 mmHg elevated for 6–10 sec after cessation of coughing. Propranolol (60 mg) and α-methyldopa (750 mg) daily in divided doses were given with no improvement in the next 16 months.

Angiography then showed hypertrophy of the left-ventricular free wall, septum and papillary muscles, as well as mitral regurgitation. There was no systolic pressure gradient between the ventricle and the aorta at rest or on exercise, but after 8 sec of coughing, a large difference in these two pressures occurred. A systolic gradient of 88 mmHg was reached, the pressure in the aorta dropped to severe hypotensive levels, with a slow return to control values (Fig. 9.1).

Autonomic nervous system vascular reflexes were intact as evidenced by increased

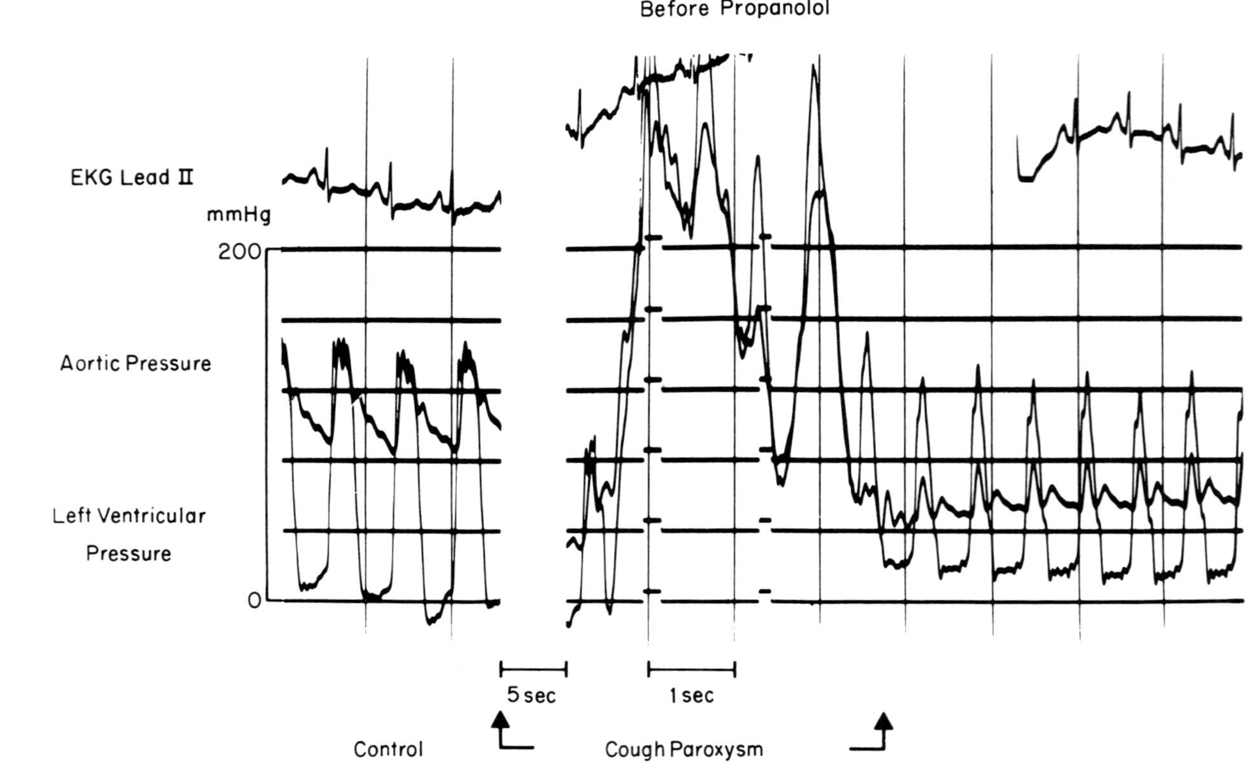

Figure 9.1 Haemodynamic response to 8 sec of cough. There is no ventricle/aorta pressure gradient in the control period. After cough the large gradient is mostly due to a reduction in aortic pressure which is at hypotensive levels and slowly returns to control levels. (Reproduced by permission of C. W. White *et al.*, 1975, and *Chest*, **68**(2): 250–253.)

peripheral resistance and reduced blood flow in the arms during leg exercise and when the lower body was subjected to negative pressure.

β-receptor blockade with i.v. propranolol reduced the ventricle/aorta pressure gradient from 88 to 6 mmHg on coughing. Although the aortic pressure still fell to hypotensive levels, the return to pre-cough levels was faster (Fig. 9.2).

Propranolol was increased to 160 mg daily for the next year with no further cough syncope. His forearm blood flow, intrathoracic and brachial arterial pressures were again studied during cough before and after i.v. propranolol. Before treatment, coughing reduced brachial artery pressure to 58/37 mmHg. Systolic pressure slowly rose to 100 mmHg in 6 sec, reaching control values in 34 sec. After propranolol, coughing reduced brachial artery pressure to 71/42 mmHg which rose to 100 mmHg systolic in 2.5 sec, and reached control levels in 13 sec. At 12 sec after coughing, forearm vascular resistance increased by 27% in the pre-treatment trial and by 59% after propranolol.

During a severe coughing attack the higher intrathoracic pressures impeded venous return and left-ventricular obstruction increased further with a decrease in aortic pressure and syncope.

Further haemodynamic information was gathered during an i.v. infusion of isoproterenol (a sympathomimetic amine, acting on β-receptors, it lowers peripheral vascular resistance and increases cardiac output by enhanced venous return plus its positive inotropic and chronotropic cardiac effects). This drug produced a marked gradient (120 mmHg) due to a major rise in ventricular pressure and a minor fall in aortic pressure. Pretreatment with propranolol reduced the isoproterenol gradient from 120 to 5 mmHg.

The conclusions suggested by this study are: (a) vigorous cough evoked reflex sympathetic stimulation; (b) as a result, myocardial contractility and the pre-existing outflow obstruction were increased; (c) when the effects of (b) were added to the decreased venous return and chamber size resulting from increased intrathoracic pressure, sustained hypotension and syncope followed.

Cough Syncope in Children

Cough syncope is uncommon in childhood. To 1970, seven cases had been recorded since the description by Charcot in 1876.

Katz (1972) reported 10 cases in asthmatic children. Pulmonary function studies showed severe bronchial spasm in these patients. It is suggested that the relative fixation of the chest in the expiratory position, plus loss of pulmonary compliance are added to the physiological events which produce the syncope on hard coughing.

Jain (1971) described cough syncope in children, two, three and six years old. Two had pertussis and one asthma. Haslam and Freigang (1985) have also reported cough syncope as a common complication of childhood asthma that may mimic epilepsy. They reported 12 children seen over a seven-year period.

Jenkins and Clarke (1981) reported an adult with whooping cough and cough syncope. In agreement with McIntosh *et al.* (1956) they suggested that the haemodynamic changes during coughing were qualitatively the same as in non-syncopal subjects, but the pressure changes were greater due to harder and more lengthy coughing in those who suffer from cough syncope.

Cough Syncope and Carotid Artery Stenosis

Strauss *et al.* (1984) reported an unusual example of cough syncope associated with marked stenoses of both common carotid arteries which improved with bypass surgery.

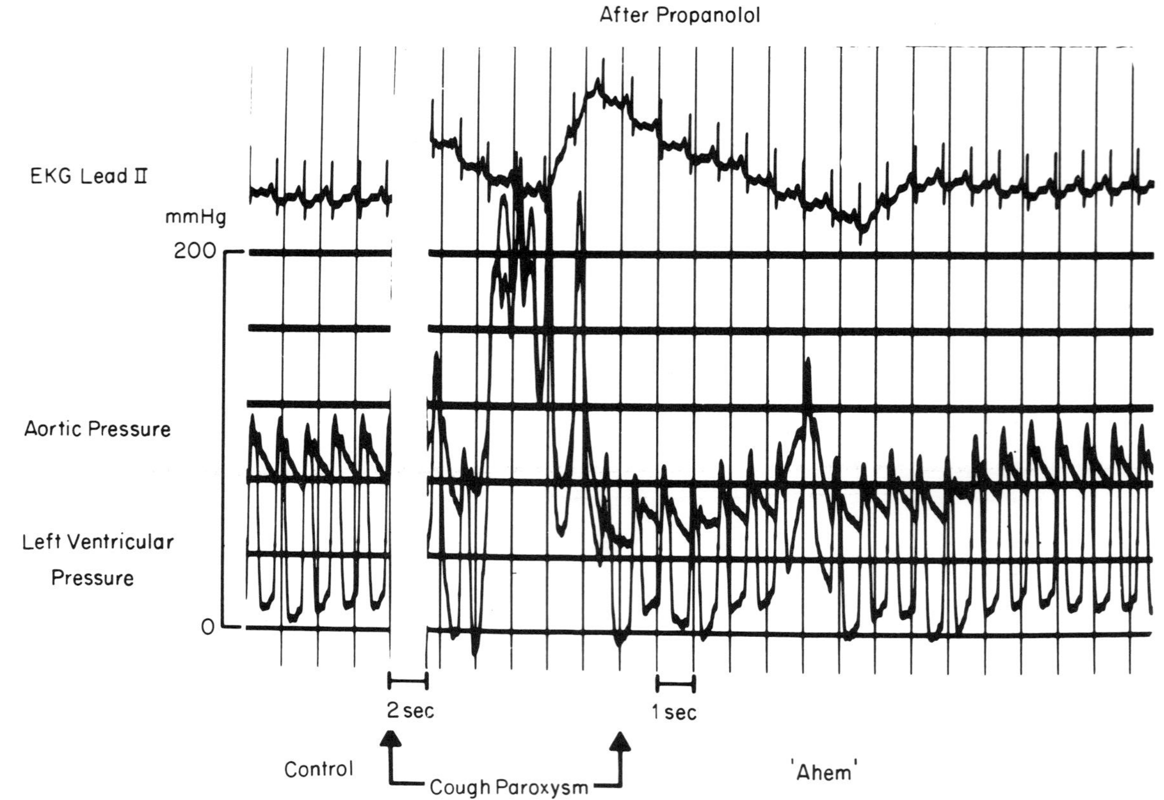

Figure 9.2 Response to 8 sec of cough after propranolol blockade. There is no ventricle-aorta gradient before or after coughing although aortic pressure fell and returned to normal more quickly. (Reproduced by permission of C. W. White *et al.*, 1975, and *Chest*, **68**(2): 250–253.)

Case study. The patient was a 51-year-old man with a six-month history of syncope after prolonged coughing. The attacks occurred daily, he smoked cigarettes, had hypertension, chronic alcoholism, angina and a previous single-vessel coronary artery bypass. Cardiac monitoring revealed normal sinus rhythm at rest and during an episode of coughing and near-syncope. Angiography showed marked stenosis of both common carotid arteries. The carotid artery obstruction was bypassed with a subclavian-to-carotid graft. The syncopal episodes were reduced but not eliminated. The procedure was done on the other side and the syncopal episodes became very rare.

Hart *et al.* (1982) and Saito *et al.* (1982) described patients with cough syncope, secondary to heart block, successfully treated by pacemaker.

Case study. The patient of Hart *et al.* was a 37-year-old female with the Holmes–Adie syndrome (tonic pupils and arreflexia). She had no heart disease, but coughing evoked prolonged atrioventricular block with ventricular asystole, syncope, and then 2:1 block before normal rhythm was restored. Pre-medication with atropine prevented the heart block and syncope. The report of Saito *et al.* concerns a 77-year-old woman with atrial fibrillation who was otherwise normal. She also developed atrioventricular block, ventricular standstill, and syncope on coughing and the sequence was prevented by atropine.

Heart block and syncope in both these patients could be evoked only by coughing. None of the other provocative tests (valsalva, carotid or eye massage, pharyngeal stimulation, methoxamine-induced hypertension, Mueller's manoeuvre—reverse valsalva, i.e. inspiration against a closed glottis) were effective.

Wenger *et al.* (1980) have described a patient with a hypersensitive carotid sinus presenting as cough syncope. Surgical denervation of the sinus resolved the symptom.

DeMaria *et al.* (1984) found the inter-ictal EEG was normal in 12 of 17 patients with cough syncope. During syncope, the EEG showed diffuse theta and delta activity as seen in other types of syncope. Although eight patients had rhythmic or clonic-like movements during the episodes, no epileptiform activity was seen.

Although cough syncope is usually a complication of chronic lung disease it exists in association with the following:

- Heart block (Hart *et al.*, 1982; Saito *et al.*, 1982)
- Idiopathic hypertrophic subaortic stenosis (White *et al.*, 1975)
- Hypersensitive carotid sinus (Wenger *et al.*, 1980)
- Carotid artery stenosis (Strauss *et al.*, 1984)
- Arnold Chiari malformation (Larsen *et al.*, 1974; Corbett *et al.*, 1976; Williams, 1980)
- Asthmatic children (Jain, 1971; Siegel and Katz, 1971; Katz, 1972)
- Syringomyelia (Hampton *et al.*, 1982)
- Syringobulbia (Jonesco-Sisesti, 1986)

PULMONARY EMBOLUS

Syncope is a recognized clinical manifestation of pulmonary emboli and has been described by Soloff and Rodman (1967). It has been reported as an initial or predominant feature in 13% of cases of acute pulmonary embolism. The mechanism is massive embolus obstructing 50% or more of the pulmonary circulation and precipitating acute cor pulmonale.

Oster and Leslie (1973) have described a patient with syncope as his only complaint. The diagnosis of pulmonary emboli was made because of a suggestive electrocardiogram and subsequent confirmation with arterial blood gas determination, lung scan and pulmonary angiography. The authors point out that an ECG suggestion of pulmonary embolus is fortuitous, as a substantial number of pulmonary emboli occur with normal ECGs.

INTENTIONAL FAINTING—'THE MESS TRICK' AND 'FAINTING LARK'

The mess trick–fainting lark consists of the victim squatting on the floor in a full knee bend and hyperventilating for 2 or 3 min. He then stands quickly, closes his mouth, pinches the nose, and tries to breath out forcefully. His friends then put their arms around his chest and squeeze. The victim then goes unconscious. Hyperventilation, followed by further diversion of an increased volume of blood into the legs (sudden upright standing after squatting), followed by a valsalva followed by a further increase in intrathoracic pressure from the squeeze by the friends should be enough to reduce anyone's cerebral blood flow to the syncopal level.

Rumball (1963) reported the case of a young man who performed such a stunt who then developed pulmonary oedema, diplopia, ataxia and dysarthria. He recovered completely.

Hyperventilation without muscular effort will reduce arterial CO_2 tension by 20 or 25 mmHg and produce constriction of cerebral veins and arteries reducing cerebral blood flow by 35% (Ruch and Fulton, 1960), while cerebral hypoxia is further augmented by a shift to the left of the oxygen dissociation curve (Bard, 1961).

The valsalva manoeuvre contributes to the situation by isolating central venous pressure from peripheral venous inflow with reduced systemic blood pressure and cardiac output.

Table 9.1 Synopsis of pulmonary disease, coughing and syncope

- Pulmonary hypertension from any cause may present with syncope on effort and primary pulmonary hypertension is more common in young women
- Sudden sustained increases in intrathoracic pressure reduce cerebral blood flow
- Hyperventilation alone almost never causes unconsciousness. It can reduce cerebral blood flow by 35% however
- Coughing can cause syncope if the cough is hard enough and long enough. It can also cause syncope if its effect is added to some pre-existing compromise of cerebral haemohydrodynamics (carotid artery occlusion, Arnold–Chiari malformation) or cardiac function (sub-aortic stenosis)
- Coughing impedes venous return and reduces cardiac output, systemic arterial pressure, and peripheral blood flow
- Atlanto-occipital junction abnormalities, such as cerebellar tonsil herniation, plus the changes from coughing or sneezing can result in syncope
- Children with cough syncope are usually asthmatics
- Syncope may be the initial and only manifestation of pulmonary embolus
- The 'mess-trick' faint is a result of reduced cerebral blood flow from the combination of (a) hyperventilation, (b) valsalva, (c) external chest compression and (d) sudden standing after being in a full knee-bend position

Cardiac output and cerebral blood flow drop below the critical level for consciousness and syncope results. The effect of rapid standing after squatting is to divert a greater proportion of cardiac output to the legs further reducing the proportion of cardiac output available for the cerebral circulation (Patterson and Warren, 1952).

Klein *et al.* (1964) studied syncope induced by deep breathing and the valsalva manoeuvre in 20 young, male, volunteer subjects, aged 18 to 29 years. They found that syncope almost always occurred at a critical level of mean arterial pressure of 51 mmHg and arterial blood CO_2 tension of 26 mmHg. Occasionally, a reduction in blood pressure alone resulted in syncope, but usually a combination of hypotension and hypocapnoea were necessary for syncope to occur. The inhalation of 100%O_2 failed to prevent or delay the onset of syncope.

The clinical features of these phenomena are summarized in Table 9.1.

REFERENCES

Bard P (1961) *Medical Physiology*, 11th Edition p. 324. St. Louis: Mosby.

Bloom N (1946) Hyperpnea test for latent coronary artery disease. *Virginia Medical Monthly* **73**: 21.

Booth RW, Ryan JM, Mellett HC, Swiss E and Netti E (1962) Hemodynamic changes associated with the valsalva manoeuver in normal men and women. *Journal of Laboratory Clinical Medicine* **59**: 275.

Brown EB (1953) Physiological effects of hyperventilation. *Physiological Review* **33**: 445.

Charcot LM (1876) *Gaz. Med. Fr. (Paris)* **5**: 588.

Charcot LM (1876) *Compt Rend. des Seance Mem. Soc. Biol.* **3**: 336–337.

Corbett JJ, Butler AB and Kaufman B (1976) 'Sneeze syncope,' basilar invagination in Arnold Chiari Type I malformation. *Journal of Neurology, Neurosurgery and Psychiatry* **39**: 381–384.

Corson WA (1970) Cough syncope. *Minnesota Medicine* **53**(1): 43.

Daly I, Ludany G, Todd A and Verney EB (1937) Sensory receptors in pulmonary vascular bed. *Quarterly Journal of Experimental Physiology* **27**: 123–146.

DeMaria AA, Westmoreland BF and Sharbroug FW (1984) EEG in cough syncope. *Neurology (Cleveland)* **34**: 371–374.

Dobkin BH (1978) Syncope in the adult Chiari abnormality. *Neurology* **28**: 718–720.

Dressler W (1952) Effort syncope as an early manifestation of primary pulmonary hypertension. *American Journal of Medical Sciences* **223**: 131–142.

Hampton F, Williams B and Loizou LA (1982) Syncope as a presenting feature of hindbrain herniation with syringomyelia. *Journal of Neurology, Neurosurgery and Psychiatry* **45**: 919–922.

Harrison TR, Calhoun JA, Cullen GE, Wilkins WE and Pilcher C (1932) Studies in congestive heart failure. XV. Reflex versus chemical factors in the production of rapid breathing. *Journal of Clinical Investigation* **11**: 133.

Hart G, Oldershaw PJ, Cull RE *et al.* (1982) Syncope caused by cough induced complete atrioventricular block *Pace* : 564–566.

Haslam RHA and Freigang B (1985) Cough syncope mimicking epilepsy in asthmatic children. *Canadian Journal of Neurological Sciences* **12**(1), 45–47.

Jain AM (1971) Cough syncope. *Indian Journal of Pediatrics* **38**: 434–435.

Jenkins P and Clarke SW (1981) Cough syncope: a complication of adult whooping cough. *British Journal of Diseases of the Chest* **75**: 311–313.

Jonesco–Sisesti N (1986) Syringobulbia: A contribution to the pathophysiology of the brainstem. Translated into English by RT Ross. New York: Praeger Publishers.

Katz RM (1972) Cough syncope in children with asthma. *The Journal of Pediatrics* **77**(1): 48–51.

Kerr A and Eich RH (1961) Cerebral concussion as a cause of cough syncope. *Archives of Internal Medicine* **108**: 248–252.

Kety SS and Schmidt CF (1946) The effect of active and passive hyperventilation on cerebral blood flow, cerebral oxygen consumption, cardiac output, and blood pressure of normal young men. *Journal of Clinical Investigation* **25**: 1.

Klein LJ, Saltzman AJ, Heyman A and Sieker HO (1964) Syncope induced by the valsalva manoeuver. *American Journal of Medicine* **37**: 263–268.

Larson SJ, Sances A, Baker JB and Reigal DH (1974) Herniated cerebellar tonsils and cough syncope. *Journal of Neurosurgery* **40**(4): 524–528.

McIntosh HD, Estes EH and Warren JV (1956) The mechanism of cough syncope. *American Heart Journal* **52**: 70–82.

Oster MW and Leslie B (1973) Syncope and pulmonary embolus. *Journal of the American Medical Association* **224**(5): 630.

Parin VV (1947) Medical research in the USSR. *American Review of Soviet Medicine* **4**: 292.

Patterson JL and Warren JV (1952) Mechanics of adjustment in the cerebral circulation upon assumption of the upright posture. *Journal of Clinical Investigation* **31**: 653.

Patterson JL, Gannon JG and Warren JR (1951) Use of continuous oxymetric technique in the study of cerebral circulation. *American Journal of Medicine* **11**: 5.

Pederson A, Sandoe E, Hvidberg E and Schwartz M (1966) Studies on the mechanism of tussive syncope. *Acta Medica Scandinavica* **179**(6): 653–661.

Ruch TC and Fulton JF (1960) *Medical Physiology and Biophysics.* Philadelphia: W.B. Saunders.

Rumball A (1963) Pulmonary edema with neurological symptoms after the fainting lark and mess trick. *British Medical Journal* No. 5349: 80–83.

Saito D, Matsuno S, Matsushita K, Takeda H, Hyodo T, Haraoka S, Watanabe A and Nagashima H (1982) Cough syncope due to atrioventricular conduction block. *Japanese Heart Journal* **23**(6): 1015–1020.

Sharpey-Schafer EP (1953) The mechanism of syncope after coughing. *British Medical Journal* **2**: 860–863.

Siegel SC and Katz RM (1971) Cough syncope. *Journal of Allergy* **47**(6): 346.

Skolnick JL and Dines DE (1969) Tussive syncope. *Minnesota Medicine* **52**(10): 1609–1613.

Soloff LA and Rodman T (1967) Acute pulmonary embolism. II. Clinical. *American Heart Journal* **74**: 710–724.

Strauss MJ, Longstreth WT and Thiele BL (1984) A typical cough syncope. *Journal of the American Medical Association* **251**(13): 1731.

Wayne HH (1958) Clinical differentiation between hypoxia and hyperventilation. *Journal of Aviation Medicine* **29**: 307.

Wenger TL, Dohrmann ML, Strauss HC *et al.* (1980) Hypersensitive carotid syndrome manifested as cough syncope. *Pace* **3**: 332–339.

White CW, Zimmerman TJ and Ahmad M (1975) Idiopathic hypertrophic subaortic stenosis presenting as cough syncope. *Chest* **68**(2): 250–253.

Williams B (1980) Cough headache due to craniospinal pressure dissociation. *Archives of Neurology* **37**: 226–230.

10

Oesophageal Syncope

SWALLOW SYNCOPE

Syncope associated with swallowing is a rare disease. According to Guberman and Catching (1986) there were only 29 reported examples up to the time of publication of their paper.

Almost all patients with swallowing syncope have pathology which is oesophageal, cardiac, or both. It is similar to carotid sinus syncope in that both diseases are more common in the presence of cardiac disease or cardiac conduction disorders.

The mechanism of syncope depends on impulse within the territories of the glossopharyngeal or vagus nerves being transmitted to the nucleus of the tractus solitarius and thence to the dorsal nucleas of the vagus, to medullary sympathetic vasodepressor centres and probably to higher autonomic centres in the hypothalamus and cortex. The resulting vagal discharge acts on the sino-atrial and atrioventricular nodes producing bradycardia and slowed atrioventricular conduction (Levin and Posner, 1972). The abnormally strong vagal discharge may cause marked sinus bradycardia, sinus arrest, asystole, or impaired atrioventricular conduction with heart block and nodal or ventricular escape beats (Lown and Levine, 1961; Sigler, 1963).

Digitalis Toxicity and Cardiac Abnormalities

Guberman and Catching (1986) reported a 62-year-old man with episodes of unconsciousness or light-headedness while eating. They were more marked if he was eating quickly and taking large mouthfuls. His barium swallow was normal except for mild reflux and marked reduction in peristalsis in the lower third of the oesophagus. His EEG was normal and an ECG revealed a heart rate of 60/min with first-degree heart block. Monitoring revealed brief periods of second-degree block type II. Digoxin level was 2.8 ng/ml (therapeutic range is 1–2 ng/ml). During EEG and ECG monitoring while eating peanut butter, he had three episodes of light-headedness associated with a heart rate of 30 and second-degreee heart block. The EEG remained normal. The digoxin was discontinued and there were no syncopal attacks in the next two years.

The most common cardiac abnormalities associated with swallow syncope are ischaemic heart disease, inferior infarction and heart block. The arrhythmias provoked by swallowing which may lead to syncope include various degrees of atrioventricular (AV) block, nodal or sinus bradycardia, ventricular asystole and atrial fibrillation (Kalloor *et al.*, 1977).

Wik and Hillestad (1975) described a 43-year-old man with a previous history of rheumatic heart disease with the sick sinus syndrome, who also had AV block while swallowing carbonated liquids. He was treated with a demand pacemaker. His oesophagus was apparently normal. Gold (1977) also reported a case of swallowing syncope with second-degree AV block and relief with a pacemaker.

There are two other reports in which digitalis was a contributing factor (Lichstein and Chadda, 1972; Armstrong *et al.*, 1985). The mechanism is partly the vagotonic effect of digitalis producing an AV conduction block, particularly with pre-existing conduction abnormalities.

The His bundle recordings while swallowing described by Lichstein and Chadda revealed periods of Mobitz Type II atrioventricular block. When the digitalis was discontinued, swallowing no longer caused syncope or the electrophysiological block.

Diffuse Oesophageal Spasm

Guberman and Catching (1986) reported the following case.

> *Case study.* A 62 year-old-woman had a two-year history of unconsciousness with meals, occurring once or twice a month. The aura was a brief hot sensation followed by a syncopal attack and recovery in 10 sec. There was no preceding dysphagia, choking or throat pain. The attacks occurred at the beginning of a meal, with liquids or solids, and were rare with breakfast. She had no other cardiac or gastrointestinal symptoms. Her heart was normal on examination. EEG and ECG telemetry while eating was normal. Oesophagoscopy was normal. Oesophageal manometry revealed abnormally high pressure in the upper and lower oesophagus during swallowing. Inflation of an oesophageal balloon 35 cm distal to her lower lip induced spontaneous high-pressure oesophageal contractions, nausea and light-headedness. Initially, there was first, and then briefly, second-degree heart block. Blood pressure did not fall. On propantheline bromide 45 min before meals, she had only four attacks in the next four years.

Bortolotti *et al.* (1982) also reported high oesophageal pressures and peristaltic abnormalities associated with AV block on swallowing.

Alstrup and Pedersen's (1973) patient had syncope on swallowing secondary to diffuse oesophageal spasm. The patient, a 64-year-old woman, developed precordial pain on swallowing, an abnormally high intraluminal oesophageal pressure and atrioventricular block. Oesophagomyotomy plus repair of a hiatus hernia abolished the attacks. Studies during the episodes revealed bradycardia as well as transient AV block.

Cold and Hot Food

Brick *et al.* (1978) reported a 51-year-old man with no symptoms or signs of disease who collapsed on swallowing a cold drink. A similar event had occurred three years earlier. The attacks could be reproduced by drinking cold water and an ECG at the same time showed AV block with 4.6 sec asystole. Putting the patient's hand in cold water produced no change and the swallowing response could be prevented by the previous administration of 0.6 mg atropine. Swallowing water at room temperature had no effect.

There are many other reports of reflex syncope on drinking cold liquids: Foster (1975), Morris (1975), Rainford (1972), Kopald (1964) and Sapru *et al.* (1971). An interesting editorial in the *Lancet* (1964) briefly reviews the subject, starting with a case reported in 1764.

Kunis *et al.* (1985) described a case of deglutition syncope with AV block selectively induced only by hot food or liquid.

Oesophageal Stretching

Fainting on swallowing is not always related to obvious pathology of the oesophagus, heart, or digitalis.

Sapru *et al.* (1971) reported the following case.

> *Case study.* A 29-year-old female had attacks of blurred vision, light-headedness and fainting on swallowing. The size, consistency or temperature of the material swallowed was immaterial and the symptoms were worse when standing. An ECG while swallowing showed episodic AV block with a normal and persistent sinus rate and no escape rhythm. During Phase IV of the valsalva manoeuvre (the hypertensive over-shoot and bradycardia after re-breathing), the sinus rate slowed. These changes were abolished by the intravenous administration of atropine sulphate. Clinical examination and a pulmonary arteriogram as well as aortogram, visualization of the left atrium and left ventriculogram, were normal. Carotid sinus or eye pressure, or somatic pain did not change her ECG nor did gargling or swallowing air. Oesophageal mobility was normal and barium swallow in all positions was normal. Inflated balloon studies of the oesophagus showed that the cardiac abnormality could be elicited from the segment of the oesophagus between T5 and T9 vertebral bodies. An attempt at oesophageal anaesthesia did not change the reflex. Because of the difference in response to vagal stimulation during Phase IV of the valsalva manoeuvre and that produced by swallowing, it was thought that the efferent impulses in the swallowing reflex might be carried by one vagus only. Unilateral vagal blocks were carried out on the two sides with lignocaine. The blocks were effective but failed to abolish the reflex. The affected segment of the oesophagus was stripped of all branches of the vagus and sympathetic nerves and the reflex was abolished.

An example of cardiac arrhythmia on swallowing due to incoordinate peristaltic activity of the oesophagus was reported by Kalloor *et al.* (1977).

Oesophageal Diverticulum and Other Diseases

Weiss and Ferris (1934) studied a patient with syncope precipitated by swallowing food. He had a traction diverticulum of the oesophagus. When this was distended by a rubber balloon atrial/ventricular dissociation of the heart and syncope occurred. Release of pressure in the balloon prompted the return of normal sinus rhythm and he recovered consciousness.

Distension of the oesophagus in normal control subjects and in patients with syncope due to a hypersensitive carotid sinus reflex failed to induce fainting or a change in cardiac rhythm. Epinephrine and ephedrine in doses which did not change the blood pressure and only changed the heart rate slightly abolished the symptom, although pressure on the diverticulum continued to induce complete heart block. Atropine abolished the symptom as well as the heart block. Paralysis of either of the vagus sheaths in the neck with procaine hydrochloride also abolished the fainting and the heart block. There are other reports of mid-oesophageal diverticula with distension of the distal third of the oesophagus, and in each of these, balloon inflation in the area of the diverticulum produced AV block (Correll and Lindert, 1949; James, 1958). The responses were blocked by atropine and some of these patients were receiving digitalis.

The patient of Trujillo and Spero (1974), aged 54 years, had a sliding hiatus hernia, oesophageal stricture, dysphagia, and complete heart block and loss of consciousness on swallowing. Atropine prevented the episodes.

HEAD AND NECK AND OTHER CANCERS

Syncope secondary to head and neck tumours has been attributed to a carotid sinus reflex from pressure or invasion of the carotid sinus, sinus nerve or glossopharyngeal nerve by tumour. The tumour may evoke an afferent discharge in the damaged nerve or lead to ephaptic conduction between efferent and afferent fibres. Spontaneous generation of impulses and ephaptic conduction between motor and sensory nerves has been documented in experimentally damaged nerve. Demyelinated nerves necessary for ephaptic conduction have been demonstrated in cases of syncope in head and neck cancer (Epstein and Shaw, 1957; Levin and Posner, 1972), in cases of glossopharyngeal neuralgia, and in two of the autopsied cases reported by Macdonald *et al.* (1983). A simple schema suggesting the mechanism of syncope by Macdonald is shown in Fig. 10.1.

Macdonald *et al.* reported 17 patients with syncope associated with head and neck cancer. The tumours were in the mouth in seven, the larynx in six, nasopharynx in three, and parotid gland in one, and involved cervical lymph nodes at diagnosis in twelve. Sixteen of their patients had radical neck dissections, 12 radiation therapy and recurrent carcinoma was present in 16. The spells resolved spontaneously in four, improved with treatment in 11 and continued in two. The syncope was spontaneous in 15, and invoked only by suctioning or carotid sinus massage in two. Suctioning also produced attacks in four others. Acute, severe, unilateral neck pain preceded the syncope in eleven. Sixteen patients has profound bradycardia and hypotension during most spells but 10 had syncope with hypotension only. Seizure activity accompanied the syncope in eight.

Anticholinergics improved seven out of 12, carbamazepine two out of five, carotid ligation one, and intracranial section of the glossopharyngeal nerve one. Local radiation may have helped four out of 10. Cardiac pacing was ineffective in three out of three with a pure vasodepressor syncope. Autopsy in two showed tumour involving the glossopharyngeal and vagus nerves.

Levin and Posner (1972) described a patient with swallow syncope following radiation of neck and mediastinum for lung cancer. At autopsy, demyelination of the vagus nerve and infiltration of the glossopharyngeal nerve with metastatic tumour was found.

Carcinoma of the Oesophagus

Tomlinson and Fox (1975) reported a 74-year-old man with syncopal episodes occurring only while eating or drinking. Monitoring revealed sinus bradycardia (as slow as 15/min) and on one occasion sinus arrest for 6 sec. Atropine before a meal prevented the episodes. A large distal oesophageal dilatation was present containing a carcinoma. Resection of the carcinoma completely relieved the syncope.

Their review of the literature from 1906 to 1973 included data on 14 similar patients. Six of these had AV block, two had complete heart block, one had sinus arrest, two had ventricular asystole, one with atrial fibrillation, and two had sinus bradycardia.

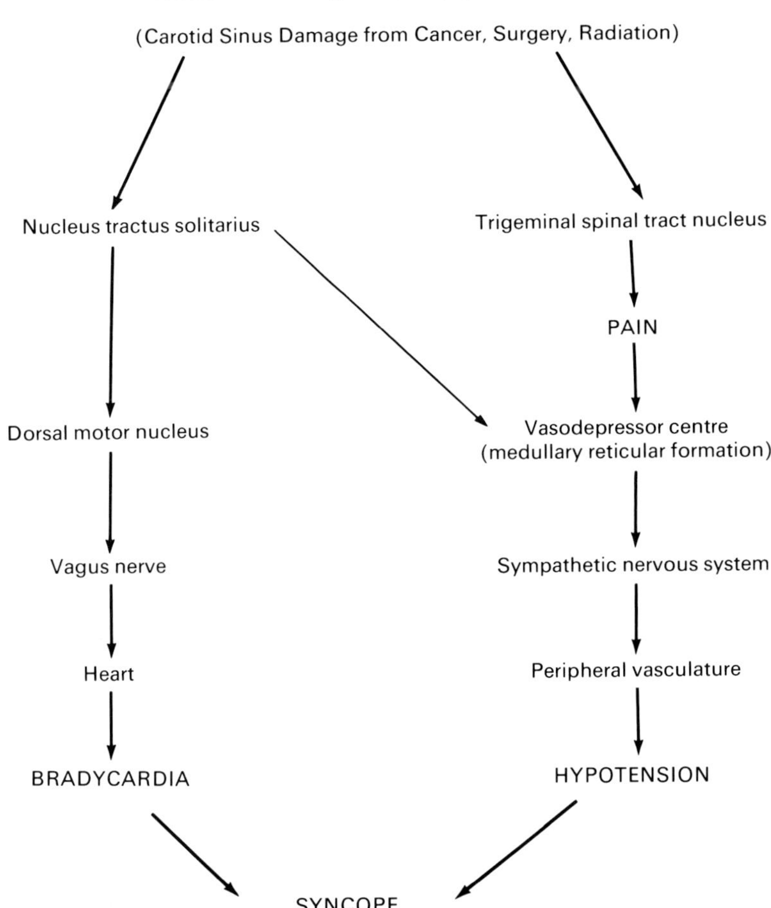

Figure 10.1 Suggested mechanism of syncope in head and neck cancer. (Reprinted by permission of J.B. Posner and Martinus Nijhoff Publishing. From D. R. Macdonald *et al.*, *Journal of Neuro-oncology*, 1983, **1**: 257–267.)

Waddington *et al.* (1975) reported a similar case with carcinoma at the junction of the middle and lower third of the oesophagus. Resection of the carcinoma stopped the attacks.

POST-PRANDIAL SYNCOPE

Fainting after eating, particularly in the elderly, is relatively common. It was a separate category in Fisher's classification of syncope (1979) and assessed by Lipsitz *et al.* (1983). They evaluated the effects of a meal on blood pressure and heart rate in elderly institutionalized patients (mean age 87 years) with and without syncope, and in young normal subjects. Pulse and blood pressure were measured before a meal and up to 60 min afterwards. By 35 min, mean systolic blood pressure had declined a maximum of 25 ± 9 mmHg in 10 elderly subjects without syncope (all sitting). The level then stabilized. There were no changes in blood pressure in 11 young subjects or elderly subjects not given a meal. The expected increase in heart rate was minimal in the elderly, indicating defective baroreflexes. This suggests that post-prandial reductions in blood pressure may predispose the elderly to symptomatic hypotension and syncope.

Robertson *et al.* (1981) studied a younger population (54–74 years of age) with idiopathic orthostatic hypotension and also observed a significant decrease in supine systolic blood pressure 15–30 min after the start of a meal.

This inadequate heart-rate response to a drop in blood pressure after eating is similar to the blunted baroreceptor response to other hypotensive stimuli such as upright posture (White, 1980), lower body negative pressure (Collins, 1980) and nitroprusside infusions (Minaker *et al.*, 1980). These have all been demonstrated in otherwise healthy elderly subjects.

Splanchnic pooling contributes to the hypotension and in addition there is evidence that insulin in response to ingested glucose further blunts the baroreceptor function particularly in the presence of cerebrovascular disease. In patients with autonomic nervous system disease, oral glucose and exogenous insulin interfere with baroreceptor mechanisms (Appenzeller and Goss, 1970; Page and Watkins, 1976).

Further, Rowe *et al.* (1981) and Minaker *et al.* (1982) have shown a different response to glucose and insulin infusions in young, as opposed to old, non-obese, men. The young had a significant increase in norepinephrine and mean arterial pressure while there was no change in norepinephrine and a decrease in mean arterial pressure in the old. A drop in blood pressure in the elderly after eating may be partly a failure of sympathetic nervous system activation in response to insulin.

Bannister *et al.* (1984) studied six patients with post-prandial hypotension and idiopathic autonomic failure and six controls. They assessed blood pressure, heart rate, plasma noradrenaline (NA), and adrenaline (A), and plasma renin activity as well as haematocrit, osmolarity, sodium, potassium and glucose in venous blood.

In the patients with autonomic failure, blood pressure fell within 15 min of eating, from 141(± 19)/77(± 9) to 102(± 24)/62(± 13) mmHg. It was lowest 1 h after eating and remained depressed for 3 h. The controls had no change in blood pressure, and neither group had a change in pulse.

Plasma NA levels were lower in the autonomic failure group at the start (0.56 ± 0.34 versus 105 ± 0.15 nmol/litre) and remained unchanged. The NA levels in the control patients changed after 1 h from 0.62 ± 0.4 to 1.44 ± 0.27 nmol/litre.

There were no changes in plasma adrenaline, haematocrit, osmolarity or sodium. The changes in potassium, plasma renin activity and glucose were similar in the two groups.

All the patients with autonomic failure had a substantial and prolonged post-prandial fall in blood pressure. The impaired autonomic reflex activity was shown by the absence of a rise in plasma NA and A and the unchanging heart rate. Stable haematocrit and osmolarity excluded significant loss of intravascular fluid into the gut. In autonomic failure, post-prandial hypotension is probably secondary to splanchnic vasodilatation, without the normal compensating sympathetic activity.

EATING EPILEPSY

Swallowing syncope can appear similar to eating epilepsy (Cirignotta *et al.*, 1977; Ahuja *et al.*, 1980). Like other kinds of syncope, a few tonic postures or clonic jerks may occur with swallow syncope particularly if the patient stays upright after losing consciousness, and this may erroneously suggest a seizure disorder.

Eating epilepsy is a rare form of reflex epilepsy and occurs with chewing and swallowing of solids but apparently not liquids. It is usually either a complex partial seizure or generalized and the generalization is often secondary. Patients with this disease usually have seizures at times not associated with meals. Although swallow syncope occurs with eating or drinking, it may be precipitated by swallowing only hot or cold liquids or only solids (Brick *et al.*, 1978; Armstrong *et al.*, 1985). Patients with eating epilepsy do not have coincidental oesophageal or cardiac abnormalities and do have inter-ictal EEG abnormalities. Video monitoring of EEG plus ECG during eating may resolve the diagnosis.

GLOSSOPHARYNGEAL NEURALGIA

In 1942, Riley *et al.* first reported that glossopharyngeal neuralgia could be associated with cardiac arrest, peripheral vasodilatation and syncope, often leading to generalized seizures. The mechanism of the cardiovascular disturbance is similar to hypersensitive carotid sinus syncope. Both are ameliorated or stopped by atropine sulphate and cured by intracranial section of the glossopharyngeal nerve.

The ninth cranial nerve carries afferent fibres from both the carotid sinus and the postero-pharyngeal wall. The pain is most common in the tonsillar area, faucial region, back of the tongue, and radiates to the front of the neck and ear on the same side. Sometimes the pain may be localized over the ear. It is spontaneous or precipitated by stimulation or movement of the oro-pharynx during chewing, swallowing, coughing, sneezing, yawning and talking. At times the pain is not paroxysmal. Not all food items will precipitate pain as the attacks may be initiated only by salty, bitter or lemon tasting food. The patient may provoke an attack with his own saliva or the pain can be spontaneous. Sudden loss of consciousness with pain in the throat prior to syncope is the distinguishing feature (Garretson and Elvidge, 1963; Khero and Mullins, 1971; Jamshidi and Masroor, 1976). Not all patients with glossopharyngeal neuralgia will have syncope, but most do.

The patient of Garretson and Elvidge (1963) could induce the pain by holding food or liquids in her mouth or by swallowing solids or liquids and it inevitably occurred if she swallowed cold water. She had some spontaneous pain. Lidocaine applied over the posterior pharynx blocked the syncope although not the pain on drinking cold water.

The patient of Khero and Mullins (1971) also had spontaneous pain. Further, glossopharyngeal neuralgia is not always described as painful. Reddy *et al.* (1987) reported a patient with a spontaneous 'tickle' on the side of her throat followed by syncope and a seizure. It also occurred with eating. Monitoring revealed asystole at the moment of the tickle, slow and then flat EEG, and unconsciousness. The attacks stopped after installation of a pacemaker.

Investigations of patients with swallow syncope should include upper gastrointestinal radiology, cine-oesophageal studies, oesophagoscopy, oesophageal manometry, mediastinal radiographic studies, ECG monitoring during eating, drinking, cold and hot liquids or oesophageal balloon inflation. When the syncope clearly follows or accompanies glossopharyngeal or trigeminal neuralgia consideration should be given to the possibilty of an aberrant posterior fossa vessel. This is a more common cause for these conditions than was once thought.

Management is difficult. De-afferentation of the oesophagus is usually unsuccessful. A permanent pacemaker has been recommended as the treatment of choice. In the absence of cardiac pathology anticholinergic agents may work, although the side-effects are considerable (Bortolloti *et al.*, 1982; Guberman and Catching, 1986).

Tolman and Ashworth (1971) relieved the syncope by dilatation of an oesophageal stricture.

Riley *et al.* (1942) reported several cases in which pharyngeal cocainization stopped the attacks of pain and cardiac arrest for up to 3 h. Intravenous atropine prevented the asystole but did not influence the pain, while intracranial section of the ninth cranial nerve and superior two filaments of the tenth cranial nerve abolished further attacks.

Lennartz (1953) reported a case of glossopharyngeal neuralgia with hypotension, asystole, and several seizures and an abnormality of the styloid process on the side of the pain. He described this as a fracture, while Garretson and Elvidge (1963) considered it to be the pseudo-articulation commonly present in the anomalous ossification of the second branchial cartillage.

Thomson (1954) reported a patient with throat pain plus generalized convulsion of 10 or 15 sec duration. The pulse was never less than 60 per minute and the blood pressure never fell below 120/70 mmHg. Carotid sinus compression did not reproduce the attacks. Intracranial section of the ninth cranial nerve and upper two filaments of the tenth cranial nerve prevented further attacks.

The patient of Garretson and Elvidge also had a long, prominent, styloid process on the side of the pain. This was excised and the pain was relieved for several months but recurred. At operation, the ninth cranial nerve was found, stimulated, and sectioned; neither event had any effect on cardiac rhythm. Post-operatively she was free of pain and examination revealed a reduced gag reflex and impairment of elevation of the right side of the soft palate. Appreciation of pin-prick deep within the right external auditory canal on the anterior and superior walls was decreased.

The patient of Khero and Mullins (1971) had spontaneous glossopharyngeal neuralgia. The pain, lasting less than a minute, was felt below the right ear radiating down the neck and up into the face. The attacks were in clusters lasting 1–2 weeks with remissions of 6 months to 1 year. Seven years after the start of the attacks the pain was precipitated by swallowing solids or liquids, particularly cold. Three months after this development and seven years after the onset, she was having more intense pain six to eight times a day, lasting 1–2 min, and for the first time the episodes were associated with an occasional loss of consciousness without convulsion.

An ECG recorded sinus bradycardia and arrest while she was unconscious. Atropine intravenously produced a normal sinus rate, massage of the carotid sinus produced no change, but touching the right tonsillar fossa caused pain.

A temporary demand pacemaker was inserted and she was given phenytoin. The attacks continued and were associated with bradycardia but no further syncope. She then had resection of the glossopharyngeal nerve and was well for the following year.

Anticonvulsant therapy, especially carbamazepine, has been suggested as treatment and is occasionally satisfactory.

Jamshidi and Masroor (1976) reported a case of glossopharyngeal neuralgia with cardiac syncope. The pain was initially triggered by swallowing solid foods but became spontaneous and would waken the patient from her sleep. Her ECG during an episode revealed sinus bradycardia and occasional sinus arrest. She was successfully treated with a permanent pacemaker and carbamazepine.

Taylor *et al.* (1977) reported a case of glossopharyngeal neuralgia and reviewed the literature from 1910. They found 32 other cases ranging in age from the mid-30s to mid-70s and found the disease twice as common in males as females. The pain was in the ear and face as well as the neck and not in the pharynx in five patients. Of the collected patients, 31 had syncope, 29 had bradycardia, 22 were asystolic and 17 had seizures. Two patients had seizures without an apparent cardiac mechanism. Treatment consisted of atropine which had no effect on the pain but abolished the cardiovascular abnomalities in 16 out of 21 patients, and phenytoin which stopped the pain in two out of seven patients and reduced the syncopal episodes in the same number. Carbamazepine temporarily reduced the pain in three and stopped the attacks in three, whereas a pacemaker prevented the pain in none but reduced the cardiovascular abnormalities in all. Intracranial nerve section of the glossopharyngeal and the superior two rootlets of the vagus was effective in all.

The two patients of Jacobson and Russell (1979) with glossopharyngeal neuralgia, arrhythmia, and syncope were both successfully treated with carbamazepine. Pain in the patient of Rees and Bicknell (1979) was initially controlled by carbamazepine which was then stopped. When the pain and syncope recurred, carbamazepine and atropine were ineffective.

Microvascular Decompression of Ninth and Tenth Cranial Nerves

Tsuboi *et al.* (1985) reported a case of glossopharyngeal neuralgia and cardiac syncope successfully treated with microvascular decompression. The patient had episodic left-sided pharyngeal pain on eating or swallowing. Relief was obtained with carbamazepine. After three years the medication was ineffective. Posterior fossa exploration showed that the left glossopharyngeal and vagus nerves were compressed by the posterior inferior cerebellar artery. Microvascular decompression resulted in relief of the neuralgia, syncope and seizures.

Carcinoma of the Pharynx

The patient of Roa and Krupin (1981) with epidermoid carcinoma of the left nasopharynx presented as glossopharyngeal neuralgia and syncope. They emphasized the anaesthetic considerations with this tumour in this location including a pre-operative demand pacemaker, continuous cardiac intraoperative monitoring, and topical anaesthesia of the oropharynx to avoid precipitation of asystole during laryngoscopy and tracheal intubation.

Kim *et al.* (1985) reported another patient with glossopharyngeal neuralgia caused by a carcinoma in the hypopharynx. The pain and episodic hypotension were relieved initially by carbamazepine. A pacemaker did not prevent the hypotension with each episode. Carbamazepine was restarted and controlled the pain, bradycardia and hypotension (another example of central sympathetic vasodepressor response?).

Glossopharyngeal Neuralgia and Disturbances of Sympathetic Function

The patient of Dykman *et al.* (1981) had metastatic laryngeal carcinoma, glossopharyngeal neuralgia and syncope. The syncope appeared to be due to hypotension, as treatment of the bradyarrhythmia failed to prevent the hypotension and syncope and carbamazepine failed to prevent the pain. The symptoms were relieved with section of the glossopharyngeal nerve and upper two rootlets of the vagus.

In this patient the hypotension was not attributable to the bradycardia since hypotension was demonstrated during cardiac pacing and during tachycardia following the use of atropine. Hypotension without bradycardia suggests a decrease in vascular resistance and/or a decrease in venous preload, assuming myocardial contractility is stable. Sympathetic vasoconstrictor tone diminution could decrease arteriolar resistance and venous preload (Abboud *et al.*, 1976).

Norepinephrine responses were blunted during the hypotensive episodes compared to the brisk response during postural stress. This fact plus the initial decrease in plasma norepinephrine during the hypotensive episodes suggests that sympathetic vasoconstriction was inhibited during this patient's paroxysms.

Stimulation of the carotid sinus nerve (in animals) reduces the discharge frequency of sympathetic nerves (Haeusler, 1973). As the glossopharyngeal nerve contains the afferent fibres from the carotid sinus and posterior pharynx, aberrant impulses as part of the neuralgia could produce sympathetic inhibition. In animals, if sympathetic vasoconstrictor responses are inhibited, cholinergic vasodilator pathways will produce hypotension (Eliasson *et al.*, 1951).

The adrenal secretion of epinephrine increased during the hypotension whereas sympathetic neural secretion of norepinephrine did not. This contrasts with the normal changes observed during postural stress. It is possible that during the painful paroxysmal episodes, selective inhibition of sympathetic vasoconstrictor tone occurred.

Cardiac pacemakers, atropine, and carbamazepine have major roles in the therapy of this disease although they were ineffective in this case. Glossopharyngeal nerve sectioning was required. During hypotensive episodes there was evidence of a suppressed adrenergic neural response and an intact adrenal medullary response. Recurrent hypotension in the absence of bradycardia, a suppressed norepinephrine response, and a transient pressor response to intravenous atropine suggested that the suppression of adrenergic vasoconstriction and perhaps cholinergic vasodilatation contributed to the hypotension.

Fagius *et al.* (1985) have de-afferented arterial and cardiopulmonary baroreceptors by blocking the glossopharyngeal and vagus nerves in the neck in two healthy volunteers. After the block there was a marked increase in muscle sympathetic activity accompanied by hypertension and tachycardia. It is certainly possible that the opposite situation, i.e. a burst of impulses as in glossopharyngeal neuralgia, would reduce muscle sympathetic activity resulting in hypotension and bradycardia.

Wallin *et al.* (1984) contributed more evidence that peripheral sympathetic inhibition adds to the hypotension of syncopal glossopharyngeal neuralgia. Their patient, a 72-year-old male, had pain in the right pharynx followed by syncope. The pain was evoked by swallowing, particularly cold fluids, coughing, or yawning, and there were no tactile trigger zones.

ECG monitoring revealed bradycardia and at times asystole up to 8 sec. A pacemaker was ineffective. The episodes were finally controlled with phenytoin and carbamazepine.

Sympathetic nerve recordings in this patient showed that pain attacks were associated with cessation of sympathetic vasoconstrictor bursts and a marked fall in blood pressure despite a functioning pacemaker. Pacing did not prevent the syncope, presumably because vasoconstrictor sympathetic outflow ceased, resulting in peripheral vasodilatation. The authors thought that during neuralgic syncope the site of abnormal spread of afferent impulses differs in each patient. If increased afferent activity in carotid sinus nerves usually causes only transient inhibition of sympathetic activity, either atropine or a pacemaker should prevent syncope in most cases. On the other hand, in the few patients where sympathetic inhibition is long-lasting, blood pressure will fall and syncope will occur despite the pacing.

There are two other case reports (Seitelberger and Bornschein, 1951; Thomson, 1954) in which there was no bradycardia and no asystole. Seizures, syncope and hypotension were present. Possibly these patients also had isolated peripheral vasodilatation in response to pain.

TRIGEMINAL NEURALGIA AND SYNCOPE

Kapoor and Jannetta (1984) reported the following.

> *Case study.* A 60-year-old man had trigeminal neuralgia associated with unconsciousness. In two episodes of pain he became asystolic, syncopal and convulsed. In many other episodes of pain his pulse slowed to 50/min. A demand pacemaker prevented further attacks of unconsciousness but the pain persisted. Carbamazepine was unsatisfactory because of side effects. At microvascular decompression of the trigeminal nerve, mechanical stimulation of the trigeminal nerve reduced the heart rate to 50/min and reduced the blood pressure from 140/70 to 107/60. Both returned to baseline at the end of stimulation. In the following 22 months there was no further pain, syncope, seizures or bradycardia.

Similarly, the 57-year-old man described by Hassam *et al.* (1987) had right facial trigeminal neuralgia with asystole in each attack, occurring up to nine times a week despite carbamazepine and phenytoin therapy. A demand pacemaker prevented further unconscious episodes.

The patient described by Arias (1985) also with trigeminal neuralgia, had postural syncope as well. Both were relieved by percutaneous rhizotomy. The patient became unconscious on sitting, although while supine she was normal apart from the facial pain. On sitting her pulse went from 76 to 42/min and blood pressure to 60/20 mmHg with a return to normal when lying down. The rhizotomy abolished the pain and syncopal episodes. No explanation or hypothesis was offered for the relationship of the symptoms.

SYNCOPE ON THE SIGHT OF FOOD

Drake *et al.* (1984) reported a lady with spells of unconsciousness followed by seizures when she was presented with food. Monitoring revealed complete AV block and ventricular standstill coinciding with the symptoms. She had no oesophageal disease but had a previous myocardial infarction, known coronary heart disease, and was being treated with digoxin and

Table 10.1 Synopsis of oesophageal syncope

- Syncope on swallowing is similar to syncope on compression of the carotid sinus, i.e. both stimuli activate a reflex in which the abnormality is usually at the effector end—the cardiac-conducting tissues
- Some swallow syncope is, however, related to oesophageal pathology, spasm, diverticula, or carcinoma. The syncope may be related to the swallowing of precise foods, i.e. only hot, cold, sour, liquids or salty food, provoke the syncope
- Patients with carcinoma of head and neck may have as an added burden syncope on swallowing, syncope with pain or suctioning of the oro-pharynx
- Post-prandial syncope is hypotensive, usually without a compensatory tachycardia, and a manifestation of slow or absent vasomotor reflexes in some elderly people. It is commonplace in patients with autonomic failure
- The syncope of glossopharyngeal and trigeminal neuralgia is usually due to asystole, but it may be entirely vasodepressor and not helped by cardiac pacing
- The syncope of glossopharyngeal neuralgia, oropharyngeal and oesophageal carcinoma appears to be followed by epileptic seizures more frequently than syncope from other causes

verapamil. It was not known if the sight of food precipitated salivation, gagging or unconscious swallowing. The symptoms were abolished with a pacemaker.

The clinical features of oesophageal syncope are summarized in Table 10.1.

REFERENCES

Abboud FM, Heistad DP, Mark AL and Schmid PG (1976) Reflex control of the peripheral circulation. *Progress in Cardiovascular Disease* **18**: 371–402.

Ahuja GK, Mohandas S and Narayanaswamy AS (1980) Eating epilepsy. *Epilepsia* **1**: 85–96.

Alstrup P and Pedersen SA (1973) A case of syncope on swallowing secondary to diffuse oesophageal spasm. *Acta Medica Scandinavica* **193**: 365–368.

Appenzeller O and Goss JE (1970) Glucose and baroreceptor function: effects of oral administration of glucose on baroreceptor function in cerebrovascular disease and in other disorders with baroreceptor reflex block. *Archives of Neurology* **23**: 137–146.

Arias MJ (1985) Neuralgia del trigemino tratamiento. *Rev. Clin. Esp.* **176**(8): 375–383.

Armstrong PW, McMillin DG and Simon JB (1985) Swallow syncope. *Canadian Medical Association Journal* **132**: 1281–1284.

Bannister R, Christensen NJ, DaCosta DF, Mathias CJ and Wright H (1984) Mechanisms of postprandial hypotension in autonomic failure. *Journal of Physiology* **349**: 67.

Bortolotti M, Cirignotta F and Labo G (1982) Atrioventricular block induced by swallowing in a patient with diffuse esophageal spasm. *Journal of the American Medical Association* **248**: 2297–2299.

Brick JE, Lowther CM and Deglin SM (1978) Cold water syncope. *Southern Medical Journal* **71**: 1571–1580.

Cirignotta F, Maracacci G and Lugaresi E (1977) Epileptic seizures precipitated by eating. *Epilepsia* **18**: 445–449.

Collins KJ, Exton-Smith AN, James MH and Oliver DJ (1980) Functional changes in autonomic nervous responses with ageing. *Age and Ageing* **9**: 17–24.

Correll HL and Lindert MCF (1949) Vagovagal syncope: report of a case apparently induced by digitalization. *American Heart Journal* **37**: 446–454.

Drake CE, Rollings HE, Han OZE, Heidary DH and Yeh TJ (1984) Visually provoked complete atrioventricular block: an unusual case of deglutition syncope. *American Journal of Cardiology* **53**(9): 1408–1409.

Dykman TR, Montgomery EB, Gerstenberger PD, Zeiger HE, Clutter WE and Cryer PE (1981) Glossopharyngeal neuralgia with syncope secondary to tumor. *American Journal of Medicine* **71**(1): 165–168.

Editorial (1964) *Lancet*, December 28, 1553–1554.

Eliasson S, Folkow B, Lindgren P and Unvas B (1951) Activation of sympathetic vasodilator nerves to the skeletal muscle in the cat by hypothalamic stimulation. *Acta Physiologica Scandinavica* **23**: 331–351.

Epstein SS and Shaw HJ (1957) Metastatic cancer of the larynx as a cause of carotid sinus syndrome. *Cancer* **10**: 933–937.

Fagius J, Wallin BG, Sundlof G, Nerhed C and Englesson S (1985) Sympathetic outflow in man after anaesthesia of the glossopharyngeal and vagus nerves. *Brain* **108**: 423–438.

Fisher CM (1979) Syncope of obscure nature. *Canadian Journal of Neurological Sciences* **6**: 7–20.

Foster H (1975) Syncope after a cold drink. *Lancet* **1**(7906): 577.

Garretson HD and Elvidge AR (1963) Glossopharyngeal neuralgia with asystole and seizures. *Archives of Neurology* **8**: 26–31.

Gold S (1977) Swallowing syncope. *Acta Medica Scandinavica* **201**: 585–586.

Guberman A and Catching J (1986) Swallow syncope. *Canadian Journal of Neurological Sciences* **13**: 267–269.

Haeusler G (1973) Central adrenergic neurones in the control of blood pressure. In *Frontiers in Catecholamine Research. Third International Catecholamine Symposium, University of Strasbourg* (Ed E Usdin and SH Snyder) pp. 879–881. New York: Pergamon Press.

Hassam AB, Abindar EG, Goldhammer EI and Malouf S (1987) Complete heart block and trigeminal neuralgia. *Neurology* **37**: 1089–1090.

Jacobson RR and Russell RWR (1979) Glossopharyngeal neuralgia with cardiac arrhythmia: a rare but treatable cause of syncope. *British Medical Journal* **1**(6160): 379–380.

James AH (1958) Cardiac syncope after swallowing. *Lancet* **1**: 771–772.

Jamshidi A and Masroor MA (1976) Glossopharyngeal neuralgia with cardiac syncope. Treatment with a permanent pacemaker and carbamazepine. *Archives of Internal Medicine* **136**: 843–845.

Kalloor GJ, Singh SP and Collis JL (1977) Cardiac arrhythmias on swallowing. *American Heart Journal* **93**(2): 235–238.

Kapoor WN and Jannetta PJ (1984) Trigeminal neuralgia associated with seizure and syncope. *Journal of Neurosurgery* **61**: 594–595.

Khero BA and Mullins CB (1971) Cardiac syncope due to glossopharyngeal neuralgia. Treatment with a transvenous pacemaker. *Archives of Internal Medicine* **128**: 806–808.

Kim SS, Lal R and Ruffy R (1985) Bradycardia and vasodepressive syncope secondary to glossopharyngeal neuralgia from hypopheryngeal tumor. *American Heart Journal* **109**(5): 1101–1102.

Kopald HH (1964) Vasovagal syncope—report of a case associated with diffuse esophageal spasm. *New England Journal of Medicine* **271**: 1238.

Kunis RL, Garfein OB, Pepe AJ and Dwyer EM (1985) Deglutition syncope and atrioventricular block, selectively induced by hot food and liquid. *American Journal of Cardiology* **55**(5): 613.

Lennartz H (1953) as quoted by Garretson and Elvidge, *Archives of Neurology* (1963) **8**: 26–31.

Levin B and Posner JB (1972) Swallow syncope—report of a case and review of the literature. *Neurology (Minneapolis)* **22**(10): 1086–1093.

Lichstein E and Chadda KD (1972) Atrioventricular block produced by swallowing, with documentation by His bundle recordings. *American Journal of Cardiology* **29**(4): 561–563.

Lipsitz LA, Nyquist RP, Wei JY and Rowe JW (1983) Postprandial reduction in blood pressure in the elderly. *New England Journal of Medicine* **309**(2): 81–83.

Lown B and Levine SA (1961) The carotid sinus: clinical value of its stimulation. *Circulation* **23**: 766–789.

Macdonald DR, Strong E, Nielson S and Posner JB (1983) Syncope from head and neck cancer. *Journal of Neurooncology* **1**: 257–267.

Minaker KL, Rowe JW and Sparrow DE (1980) Impaired cardiovascular adaptation to vasodilatation in the elderly. *Gerontologist* **20** (part 2): 163 (abstract).

Minaker KL, Rowe JW, Young JB, Sparrow D, Pallotta JA and Landsberg L (1982) The effect of age on insulin stimulation of sympathetic nervous system activity in man. *Metabolism* **31**: 181–184.

Morris D (1975) Syncope after a cold drink. *Lancet* **1**(7906): 577.

Page MMcB and Watkins PJ (1976) Provocation of postural hypotension by insulin in diabetic autonomic neuropathy. *Diabetes* **25**: 90–95.

Rainford DJ (1972) Cold drink and syncope. *British Medical Journal* **3**: 475.

Reddy K, Hobson DE, Gomori AJ and Sutherland GR (1987) Painless glossopharyngeal 'neuralgia' with syncope. A case report and literature review (in press).

Rees JR and Bicknell PG (1979) Glossopharyngeal neuralgia with syncope. *British Medical Journal* **1**(6165): 754.

Riley HA, German WJ, Wortis H, Zahn D and Eichna L (1942) Glossopharyngeal neuralgia initiating or associated with cardiac arrest. *Transactions of the American Neurological Association* **68**: 28.

Roa NL and Krupin BR (1981) Glossopharyngeal neuralgia with syncope—anaesthetic consideration. *Anaesthesiology* **54**: 426–428.

Robertson D, Wade D and Robertson RM (1981) Postprandial alterations in cardiovascular hemodynamics in autonomic dysfunctional state. *American Journal of Cardiology* **48**(6) 1048–1052.

Rowe JW, Young JB, Minaker KL, Stevens AL, Pallotta J and Landsberg L (1981) Effect of insulin and glucose infusions on sympathetic nervous system activity in normal man. *Diabetes* **30**: 219–225.

Sapru RP, Griffiths PH, Guz A and Eisele J (1971) Syncope on swallowing. *British Heart Journal* **33**: 617–622.

Seitelberger F and Bornschein H (1951) As reported by JN St. John (1982), Glossopharyngeal neuralgia associated with syncope and seizures. *Neurosurgery* **10**(3): 380–383.

Sigler LH (1963) The cardio-inhibitory carotid sinus reflex. Its importance as a vasocardiosensitivity test. *American Journal of Cardiology* **12**: 175–183.

Taylor PH, Gray K, Bicknell PG and Rees JR (1977) Glossopharyngeal neuralgia with syncope. *Journal of Laryngology and Otolaryngology* **91**(10): 859–868.

Thomson JL (1954) Glossopharyngeal neuralgia accompanied by unconsciousness. *Journal of Neurosurgery* **11**: 511–514.

Tolman KG and Ashworth WD (1971) Syncope induced by dysphagia. Correction by esophageal dilatation. *Digestive Diseases* **16**: 1026–1031.

Tomlinson IW and Fox KM (1975) Carcinoma of the esophagus with 'swallow syncope.' *British Medical Journal* **2**(5966): 315–316.

Trujillo NP and Spero C (1974) Syncope associated with esophageal stricture. *Medical Annals of the District of Columbia* **43**(11): 553–556.

Tsuboi M, Suzuki K, Nagao S and Nishimoto A (1985) Glossopharyngeal neuralgia with cardiac syncope. A case successfully treated with microvascular decompression. *Surgical Neurology* **24**: 279–283.

Waddington JKB, Matthews HR, Evans CC and Ward DW (1975) Carcinoma of the esophagus with swallow syncope. *British Medical Journal* **3**(5977): 232.

Wallin BG, Westerberg C-E and Sundlof G (1984) Syncope induced by glossopharyngeal neuralgia: sympathetic outflow to muscle. *Neurology (Cleveland)* **234**: 522–524.

Weiss S and Ferris EB (1934) Adams–Stokes syndrome with transient complete heart block of vasovagal reflex origin. *Archives of Internal Medicine* **54**: 931–951.

White NJ (1980) Heart rate changes on standing in elderly patients with orthostatic hypotension. *Clinical Sciences* **58**: 411–413.

Wik B and Hillestad L (1975) Deglutition syncope. *British Medical Journal* **3**(5986): 747.

11

Pelvic Syncope

MICTURITION SYNCOPE

Introduction

Micturition syncope as described by Proudfit and Forteza (1959) is an episode of syncope at the start, during, end, or immediately after urination. It occurrs in men and women, is more common in the former and may occur at any age.

Kapoor *et al.* (1985) have divided the disease into a group of young (mean age 25 years) males with no evidence of any other condition, and a second group of either sex (mean age 60 years) with a host of concurrent medical problems and medications.

In younger males it appears as a rare and isolated phenomenon. Typically a 25-year-old male with no previous medical history and a normal physical examination spends the evening with friends drinking beer.

He retires at 1 a.m. somewhat intoxicated and is awakened at 2:30 a.m. by the desire to void. He has been awake on and off for the previous half hour for the same reason but has resisted getting up. Finally, he leaps out of bed, walks to the bathroom, voids a large amount while standing and on returning to bed is quickly light-headed, nauseated, and falls to the floor in a faint. He recovers in minutes, can give a good account of the episode the next day, is normal on examination, and now that he has been reminded, can remember a similar episode about two or three years earlier.

Micturition syncope occurs under other circumstances in which obvious abnormalities conducive to fainting are present. However, the above history is the common clinical story and the mechanism of the syncope is so subtle and evanescent that an understanding of the process is seldom obtained.

Donker *et al.* (1972) thought the syncope was due to a combination of orthostatic hypotension and reflexly-induced vagal bradycardia. Similarly Haldane (1969) believed that a vagal reflex originating from the bladder precipitated a cardiac dysrythmia and standstill, and this plus a poor autonomic adjustment to standing produced the syncope. Friedberg (1971) monitored a patient who on voiding less than an ounce had a progressive fall in blood pressure, a two-to-one heart block, ventricular rate of 20 and syncope. Micturition in normal subjects has no effect on blood pressure (Littler *et al.*, 1974).

Many, but not all, of the patients with micturition syncope who have been monitored and examined physiologically have been found to have postural hypotension, intermittent heart block, or other rhythm disorder or both, to explain the syncope. How micturition can compound and initiate the cardiovascular abnormality is not well understood, but the distended bladder and the rapidly emptied bladder both provide strong stimuli to the autonomic nervous system. Bladder filling for cystometric examination in two patients with apparently normal autonomic nervous systems has been reported by Godec and Cass (1981) to cause syncope.

Bladder Distension

Moore (unpublished observation, see Whitteridge, 1960) demonstrated peripheral vasoconstriction in normal subjects when intravesical pressure above 50 mmHg was produced. Carmichael *et al.* (1939) showed the same phenomenon when the duodenum was distended to pressure in excess of 30 mmHg.

Whitteridge (1960) has suggested that distension of any hollow viscus to a pressure above a critical level will result in peripheral vasoconstriction in normal subjects. He pointed out that the wave of goose flesh frequently experienced by normal persons on emptying the bladder is probably accompanied by a wave of cutaneous vasoconstriction.

Much information on the effect of bladder distension and stimulation on blood pressure has been obtained from the study of quadriplegic man.

Guttman and Whitteridge (1947) established that bladder distension in patients with complete cord lesions caused intense peripheral vasocontriction via the sympathetic fibres arising from the cord below the lesion. In low thoracic lesions, any elevation of blood pressure was controlled via carotid and aortic baroreceptor reflexes by vasodilatation of vessels with intact autonomic innervation above the lesion. In lesions above the seventh thoracic level, the number of vessels accessible to reflex vasodilatation was not adequate to counter elevation of blood pressure. Bladder distension resulted in flushing of the face, throbbing headache, and a substantial rise in blood pressure, as did instrumentation of the genito-urinary tract.

Mathias *et al.* (1976) measured blood pressure, heart rate, and plasma catecholamine levels in 16 patients with complete spinal cord transections above the level of the sympathetic outflow. Resting blood pressure, plasma norepinephrine, and epinephrine were all lower in the quadriplegics than in the normals. They induced hypertension by bladder stimulation.

Blood pressure rose from an average of 109/60 to 168/87 mmHg as a result of uninhibited sympathetic nervous activity through the isolated spinal cord. Plasma norepinephrine also rose but not above the resting levels in the normal controls.

They concluded that the severe hypertension of bladder stimulation was due to reflex discharge through the isolated spinal cord and the lack of blood pressure restraining reflexes, i.e. baroreceptor reflexes without efferent sympathetic pathways. A similar mechanism must apply to the hypertensive crises in patients with spinal anaesthetic and post-operative urinary retention and an over-distended bladder (O'Connor, 1920).

The absence of hypertension in normal man with a distended bladder is the result of active inhibition. It is possible that this baroreceptor-initiated vasodilatation and bradycardia is extended farther than needed and syncope results. The sequence in micturition syncope may be bladder contraction accompanied by vasoconstriction (and in the absence of intact baroreceptors, hypertension), followed by reflex vasodilatation, bradycardia, hypotension, and, in the right person at the right time, syncope. This resembles the mechanism of vasovagal fainting in response to fear or fright, i.e. initial rise in blood pressure and pulse followed by the normal correcting mechanism, over-correction, dilatation, hypotension, bradycardia and syncope.

Bladder Emptying

O'Connor (1920) found the blood pressure fell over 48 h after drainage of the bladder in patients with prostatic obstruction. Sudden decompression of the distended urinary bladder can cause circulatory collapse (Shaw and Young, 1924; Maclean *et al.*, 1944). The abrupt reversal of the vasodepressor effect of bladder distension may be all that is necessary to cause syncope in the standing, sleepy, micturating normal male.

Baroreceptor activity counters sympathetic activity, and after bladder empyting sympathetic excitation ceases and vasodilatation occurs (Johnson and Spalding, 1974). If baroreceptor sympathetic inhibition is prolonged, the degree of vasodilatation plus the erect posture of the voiding male may induce hypotension and a faint (Coggins *et al.*, 1964). A combination of orthostatic hypotension, cardio-inhibitory reflexes from the bladder and reflex vasodilatation may be the key features (Lukash *et al.*, 1964). Fatigue, alcohol excess and hunger, appear to be important contributing factors to micturition syncope (Lyle *et al.*, 1961).

In addition, breath-holding and/or the valsalva manoeuvre (which some men do while voiding) cause a cardiac dysrhythmia in the appropriate subject. Both manoeuvres will diminish venous return to the heart, although these alone will never raise intrathoracic pressure high enough in normal subjects to produce syncope (Sharpey-Schafer, 1953).

The detrusor muscle of the urinary bladder is supplied by the parasympathetic nervi erigentes from sacral segments 2, 3 and 4. The trigone is innervated by the sympathetic epigastric nerve. It has been suggested that the trigone helps to open the internal vesical orifice. At the start of micturition, contraction of the trigone depresses the posterior lip of the internal sphincter. Then contraction of the detrusor muscle opens the internal orifice further and the abdominal muscles contract with an increase in intra-abdominal pressure.

Haldane (1969) has postulated that micturition syncope may be an imbalance between the trigone muscles (sympathetic) and the detrusor (parasympathetic). If a strong vagal stimulus was required to contract the detrusor this same stimulus might inhibit the heart in a suitable individual. Added to this are postural hypotension plus the residual changes which occur during sleep.

Pickering (1965) observed that blood pressure falls during sleep with no change in heart rate, suggesting that the baroreceptors either do not function during sleep or have an altered afferent setting. The parasympathetic outflow which is necessary for voiding might further decrease an already low blood pressure and explain why micturition syncope occurs most often after sleep. Standing would add to the problem but is not the sole mechanism as micturition syncope can occur when the subject (either sex) is voiding while sitting.

Gastaut and Fischer-Williams (1957) have also suggested that the increased parasympathetic activity associated with micturition together with reduction of vasomotor tone and sudden assumption of the erect posture, might be important factors in micturition syncope. In addition, normal man standing perfectly motionless is hovering on the verge of circulatory collapse. Further, the response to standing quickly is a drop in blood pressure which also initiates reflex vasoconstriction.

Diseases and Situations Conducive to Micturition Syncope

Gastaut (1956), in a discussion of 200 cases of nocturnal episodes of unconsciousness, included 40 cases of syncope before, during or after micturition. While the true incidence of micturition syncope remains obscure, in the patient population seen at the School of Aerospace Medicine micturition syncope was common (Lyle *et al.*, 1961). These authors presented a detailed description of 24 cases of the syndrome.

Classically, the syncope occurred when the subject voided immediately after rising from recumbency. The loss of consciousness was abrupt, brief and recovery complete. Some adult patients report similar attacks in childhood. Most patients report the unconsciousness at the *end* of voiding.

Predisposing features were chronic fatigue, hunger, minor upper respiratory infection, some emotional distress or alcohol abuse. By far the most common predisposing factor in the report of Lyle *et al.* (1961) was the prior ingestion of alcohol in 14 of 25 episodes. In this group the results of standard ECG, double Masters exercise tolerance tests, ECG during orthostasis for 5 min, breath-holding at maximum inspiration, carotid sinus massage, positive pressure breathing against 11 mmHg, maximum breath-holding after hyperventilation while standing, tilt table consisting of 12-min upright followed by maximum breath-holding both before and after hyperventilation, were all normal.

From this study micturition syncope appears to be a disease *sui generis.* Moreover, it may be an exclusive abnormality and need not be associated with any other evidence of vasomotor instability or cardiac rhythm disorder.

Micturition Syncope and Circulatory Collapse

Lukash *et al.* (1964) studied a 20-year-old sailor with micturition syncope. He had been found on the floor after voiding and was apnoeic and cyanotic. No blood pressure or heart sound were present. After resuscitation, two further episodes of asystole occurred in the next few minutes. He recovered completely.

He had three previous faints, all after a period of recumbency, usually in the early morning hours and on standing. Two of them had been associated with micturition.

This patient had occasional orthostatic hypotension which sometimes coincided with voiding and a cardio-inhibitory reflex producing asystole. Whether these two phenomena are in any way related to bladder distension or bladder empyting is not known.

Bladder Reflex Bradycardia, Heart Block, Asystole and Hypotension

Schoenberg *et al.* (1974) reported the following.

> *Case Study.* A 68-year-old patient had syncope associated with an urge to urinate. He became unconscious when standing to void, unrelated to previous sleep or recumbency. Whenever he had the urge to urinate, if he was unable to void promptly, he became dizzy and unconscious. After a cystoscopic examination, a syncopal episode occurred. While having an electrocardiographic recording he had an urge to void and then had sinus bradycardia at 48 beats per minute and a fall in blood pressure to 90/50 mmHg. During voiding there was a period of asystole for 6 sec. On another occasion during micturition there were 8 sec of complete atrioventricular block. Carotid sinus massage and the valsalva manoeuvre produced only transient slowing of his heart rate and no rhythm change. After 0.6 mg of atropine sulphate intravenously, his pulse went from 70 to 90/min and there was then no alteration in cardiac rhythm with the onset of micturition. A permanent transvenous demand pacemaker was inserted and he was asymptomatic thereafter.

This patient is different from the usual patient with micturition syncope. He was elderly, had pre-existing cardiovascular (myocardial infarction) and urinary tract disease, and the syncope was associated with both bladder stretching and emptying.

Prozen and Litwin (1961) described three cases of post-micturition syncope. All had syncope following micturition but not during it. During the episode one patient had atrial fibrillation, a high degree of atrioventricular block, ventricular premature beats, and a heart rate of 50/min. Sinus arrest, nodal rhythm, and T-vector changes were produced in Phase IV of the valsalva manoeuvre and all were abolished by atropine. An ECG some hours after a syncope in their second patient revealed T-wave changes suggestive of injury to the postero-lateral wall, which were not substantiated. These changes were not reproduced by the two-step exercise test but were duplicated during Phase IV of the valsalva manoeuvre. Sinus arrest and nodal rhythm were also observed during the valsalva manoeuvre. A valsalva manoeuvre after a syncope in the third patient produced sinus arrest with a total escape rhythm which persisted for 15 sec. The T-vector diminished in magnitude but did not change direction. These authors suggested that cardiac standstill and subsequent arrhythmias in Phase IV of the valsalva manoeuvre is a cause of syncope following micturition in some people. (Phase IV occurs after release and is the second rise in blood pressure. This overshoot activates carotid and aortic baroreceptors and produces bradycardia and vasodilatation.)

Donker *et al.* (1972) reported the following.

> *Case study.* A 37-year-old pilot was examined with EEG and ECG during three spontaneous episodes of nocturnal micturition syncope. The recordings began when he retired and monitoring continued during sleep, waking, rising and voiding in the upright position. The fainting occurred 30 sec *after* the end of voiding and from the recordings the attacks were not epileptic and not explained by bradycardia alone. Ocular compression, the valsalva manoeuvre and carotid sinus massage had no effect.
>
> At the start of voiding, the subject's pulse increased from 72 to 130 per minute and blood pressure was 130/80 mmHg. After starting to void, the pulse decreased to 60 per minute, he complained of light-headedness, and his blood pressure was found to be 80/60 mmHg. On one of the three occasions, just before he collapsed, the ECG showed sinus bradycardia followed by a period of two-to-one atrioventricular block with a ventricular rate of 28 per minute. These authors thought that the reaction upon assuming the upright position consisted of bradycardia and heart block plus lowered peripheral resistance, and these three caused the syncope.

Kapoor *et al.* (1985) studied prospectively 33 patients who had syncope in association with micturition. Eight were healthy young males averaging 25 years of age with no history of disease and a normal examination. The remaining 25 had an average age of 60 years, and 16 of these were women. They defined micturition syncope as described by Proudfit and Forteza (1959). The 25 older patients had multiple concurrent medical problems with an average of 3.8 acute or chronic illnesses per patient and each patient was taking an average of 3.5 medications. Sixteen of these patients had a single episode and nine had recurrent episodes.

Physical examination in this group demonstrated orthostatic hypertension in 22 of 25 patients. Fourteen had been taking diuretics, two had been subjected to prolonged bed-rest post-operatively, two had had gastrointestinal bleeding, one an autonomic neuropathy, one had severe nausea and vomiting, and one had symptomatic orthostatic hypotension associated with paroxysmal atrial fibrillation. Prolonged ECG monitoring was not diagnostically useful.

Ventricular Fibrillation

Luria *et al.* (1963) described a case of micturition syncope in a 62-year-old woman. She had atrioventricular block. An ECG recorded during an attack revealed ventricular fibrillation induced by frequent premature ventricular beats. The syncope occurred in both the recumbent and sitting positions and the valsalva manoeuvre had no effect. The syndrome could be initiated by stimulation of the urethral meatus which could be rendered unresponsive by topical anaesthesia. Atropine failed to prevent the attacks. In this patients, manipulation of the urethra may have transmitted impulses via the spinal cord to cardiac sympathetics and could have stimulated one or more ventricular ectopic foci.

DEFAECATION SYNCOPE

There is some evidence from animal research suggesting that stretching or contraction of the gut stimulates vagal afferent fibres.

Iggo (1957a) isolated single unmyelinated afferent fibres in the cervical portion of the feline vagus nerve. He recorded electrical activity from the oesophagus, stomach and intestines. Distension pressure as low as 2 mmHg stimulated the most sensitive units. If distension was maintained the frequency of discharge fell slowly. The more rapid the distension the greater the initial impulse frequency. Bursts of impulses also occurred during contractions of the oesophagus, stomach and intestine, and this was unaffected by cutting open the organ. The tension receptors, located in the muscle layer, were fired by either stretch or contraction.

Using a similar technique, Iggo (1957b) demonstrated vagal afferent activity induced by stimulating alimentary mucosa by touch or by application of chemicals. Recording from isolated fibres in the sacral parasympathetic nerves, he had obtained similar results when studying bladder contractions (Iggo, 1955). The reflex mechanisms initiated by bladder distension and emptying can be triggered from similar stimuli to the bowel.

Because of the adaptive qualities of the bowel wall, pressures of the height attained in the distended bladder are rarely seen. Blood-pressure elevation from rectal distension in high level paraplegics is known and manual removal of faeces can cause a paroxysm of severe hypertension in these patients (Harvey, 1964).

Syncope following sudden evacuation of the bowel is recognized and is analogous to micturition syncope. Patients have been observed to be relatively well after a large upper gastrointestinal haemorrhage and at the time of evacuation of the large blood-containing stool, suddenly faint (Bockus, 1963). Syncope in a patient after evacuation of a large therapeutic enema is a similar situation.

Pathy (1978) reported defaecation syncope in seven female and two male patients, aged between 63 and 78 years. The syncope occurred in bouts of two to three times over a two-week period with intervals of freedom from weeks to 12 months. The common history was the urge to move the bowels in the early morning and the syncope occurred before the movement was complete. It was more common in patients who were constipated and had manual bowel evacuation or major evacuation from laxatives. The insertion of a rectal balloon while the subject was lying down, and slow inflation and rapid deflation of the balloon was performed in two patients with this syndrome. There were no changes in one patient. In the other, ventricular extrasystoles increased from an average of one per 10 ventricular complexes to three per 10 complexes. Blood pressure rose slightly on inflation and returned to the resting level within 3 min of deflation in both subjects. Five subjects with orthostatic hypotension but no history of defaecation syncope had the same balloon inflation and deflation. No changes occurred in blood pressure either before or during distension in any patient. In one patient ventricular extrasystoles developed and continued for 30 sec after deflation.

Scott and Sancetta (1950) reported the following.

> *Case study.* A 62-year-old lady had daily episodes of collapse and unconsciousness usually when having a bowel movement. Her blood pressure was 140/85 and an ECG revealed almost complete atrioventricular block with an atrial rate of 104 and ventricular rate of 52.
>
> Her attacks could also be precipitated by digital, rectal examination. The prodrome was a sudden irregularity and increase in pulse. At the start of an attack she was short of breath and faint, the radial pulse and heart sounds disappeared. Breathing was irregular, clonic convulsions with dilatation of the pupils, twitching of the face, and spasmodic movements of the arm occurred. She became cyanotic and the attack ended after $\frac{1}{2}$ to 3 min.
>
> An ECG while the patient was asymptomatic showed a sinus rhythm, a rate of 92 and intermittent intraventricular block. Most of the beats were idioventricular and multifocal. Short bursts of ventricular fibrillation were present. A cardiogram, while anal examination was performed, showed rapid ventricular activity suggesting a ventricular tachycardia or a coarse ventricular fibrillation with a ventricular rate of 300 per minute. The patient became unconscious.

RECTAL EXAMINATION AND SIGMOIDOSCOPY

Bilbro (1970) has recorded eight episodes of syncope or faintness during 2500 prostatic examinations. One patient had a brief generalized seizure and all patients turned pale and were bradycardic. Klotz (1970) has reported the same phenomenon.

Poleschuck (1970) has described a similar syncopal episode in a 30-year-old man following a prostatic examination. He also had bradycardia and had a family history of a similar abnormality in his father and paternal uncle. Cardiac arrest and three deaths have been reported in a series of 1800 sigmoidoscopies by Fletcher *et al.* (1968). The patient reported by Tizes (1981) became unconscious after rectal examination and while remaining supine.

PELVIC EXAMINATION

Menzies (1971) reported syncope following pelvic examination and also accompanying insertion of an intrauterine device. The mechanisms appear to be gross bradycardia, hypotension, and even cardiac arrest. It can be prevented or reversed by the administration of intravenous atropine.

Conrad *et al.* (1973) have reported six women with 'acute neurovascular sequelae' following intrauterine device (IUD) insertion or removal. Most were syncopal episodes with bradycardia, pallor, sweating, and if standing, unconsciousness and some seizure activity. The episodes were short-lived and there were no fatalities.

Some of the salient clinical features of reflexly-induced pelvic syncope are summarized in Table 11.1.

Table 11.1 Synopsis of pelvic syncope

- Micturition syncope occurs in either sex at the start, during, or after voiding while standing or sitting
- Micturition syncope occurs in two groups of patients:
  —young men with no disease
  —a group, aged 60 years plus, either sex, with a number of other conditions
- From the monitoring of patients who fainted while voiding the mechanism seems to be a reflex induced vagal excess of heart block, or other dysrhythmia, plus vasodilatation
- Bladder stretching and bladder emptying can induce the vasomotor changes that will lead to syncope
- The fortuitous combination of fatigue, hunger, alcohol excess, plus standing still and perhaps performing a valsalva manoeuvre account for the random and rare occurrence of micturition syncope in the healthy young male
- Syncope also occurs after defaecation, rectal examination, sigmoidscopy and pelvic examination. The mechanism seems to be bradycardia, heart block, or other arrhythmia, hypotension and collapse

REFERENCES

Bilbro RH (1970) Syncope after prostatic massage. *New England Journal of Medicine* **282**: 167–168 (letter to the Editor.

Bockus H (1963) *Gastroenterology*, p. 641. Philadelphia and London: W. B. Saunders.

Carmichael EA, Doupe J, Harper AA and McSwiney BA (1939) Vasomotor reflexes in man following duodenal distension. *Journal of Physiology (London)* **95**: 276.

Coggins CH, Lillington GA and Gray CP (1964) Micturition syncope. *Archives of Internal Medicine* **113**: 14–18.

Conrad CC, Ghazi M and Kitay DZ (1973) Acute neurovascular sequelae of intrauterine device insertion or removal. *Journal of Reproductive Medicine* **11**(5): 211–212.

Donker DNJ, Robles de Medina EO and Kieft J (1972) Micturition syncope. *Electroencephalography and Clinical Neurophysiology* **33**: 328–331.

Fletcher GF, Earnest DL, Shuford WF and Wenger NK (1968) Electrocardiographic changes during routine sigmoidoscopy. *Archives of Internal Medicine* **122**: 483–486.

Friedberg CK (1971) Syncope. Pathological physiology: differential diagnosis and treatment. (I). *Modern Concepts in Cardiovascular Disease* **40**: 55–60.

Gastaut H (1956) La syncope nocturne des hypervagotoniques, sa différenciation de 'avec le' epilepsie morphique. *Revue Neurologique* **95**: 420.

Gastaut H and Fischer-Williams EM (1957) Étude electroencephalographie chez 25 sujets enregistres pendant leur syncope. *Revue Neurologique* **95**(6): 524–527.

Godec CJ and Cass AS (1981) Micturition syncope. *Journal of Urology* **126**: 551–552.

Guttmann L and Whitteridge D (1947) Effects of bladder distension on autonomic mechanisms after spinal cord injuries. *Brain* **70**: 361–404.

Haldane JH (1969) Micturition syncope. *Canadian Medical Association Journal* **101**(12): 53–54.

Harvey P (1964) Cardiovascular reflexes of visceral origin. *Medical Journal of Australia* **2**: 416–419.

Iggo A (1955) Tension receptors in the stomach and the urinary bladder. *Journal of Physiology (London)* **128**: 593.

Iggo A (1957a) Gastrointestinal tension receptors with unmyelinated afferent fibres in the vagus of the cat. *Quarterly Journal of Experimental Physiology* **42**: 130.

Iggo A (1957b) Gastrointestinal chemoreceptors with vagal afferent fibres in the cat. *Quarterly Journal of Experimental Physiology* **42**: 398.

Johnson RH and Spalding JMK (1974) *Disorders of the Autonomic Nervous System*. London: Blackwell Scientific Publications.

Kapoor WN, Peterson JR and Karpf M (1985) Micturition syncope: a reappraisal. *Journal of the American Medical Association* **253**(6): 796–798.

Klotz PG (1970) Syncope during prostatic examination. *New England Journal of Medicine* **282**: 1046.

Littler WA, Honour NJ and Sleight P (1974) Direct arterial pressure, pulse rate and electrocardiogram during micturition and defecation in unrestricted man. *American Heart Journal* **88**: 205–210.

Lukash WM, Sawyer GT and Davies JE (1964) Micturition syncope produced by orthostasis and bladder distension. *New England Journal of Medicine* **270**(7): 341–344.

Luria MH, Abrams D, Lopez JF and Ohringer L (1963) Syncope in advanced AV block induced by micturition. *American Heart Journal* **65**: 357–360.

Lyle CB, Monroe JT, Flinn DE and Lamb LE (1961) Micturition syncope. Report of 24 cases. *New England Journal of Medicine* **265**(20): 982–986.

Maclean AE, Allen EV and Magrath TB (1944) Orthostatic tachycardia and orthostatic hypotension: defects in return of venous blood to the heart. *American Heart Association* **27**: 145–163.

Mathias CJ, Christensen NJ, Corbett JL, Frankel HL and Spalding JMK (1976) Plasma catecholamines during paroxysmal neurogenic hypertension in quadriplegic man. *Circulation Research* **39**: 204–208.

Menzies DN (1971) Syncope on pelvic examination. *British Medical Journal* No. 716: 221 (letter to the Editor).

Moore (1960) [Unpublished observation] quoted in Whitteridge D (1960).

O'Connor VJ (1920) Observations on blood pressure in cases of prostatic obstruction. *Archives of Surgery* **1**: 359–367.

Pathy MS (1978) Defecation syncope. *Age and Ageing* **7**: 233–236.

Pickering G (1965) Hyperpieses. High blood pressure without evident cause: essential hypertension. *British Medical Journal* **2**: 959–968.

Poleschuck VA (1970) Prostatic prostration. *New England Journal of Medicine* **282**: 632.

Proudfoot WL and Forteza ME (1959) Micturition syncope. *New England Journal of Medicine* **260**: 328–331.

Prozan GB and Litwin A (1961) Post-micturition syncope. *Annals of Internal Medicine* **54**: 82–89.

Schoenberg BS, Kuglitsch JF and Karnes WE (1974) Micturition syncope—not a single entity. *Journal of the American Medical Association* **229**(12): 1631–1633.

Scott RW and Sancetta SN (1950) Stokes–Adams attacks induced by rectal stimulation in a patient with complete heart block. *Circulation* **2**: 886–889.

Sharpey-Schafer EP (1953) The mechanism of syncope after coughing. *British Medical Journal* **2**: 860–863.

Shaw EC and Young HH (1924) Gradual decompression in chronic vesicle distension. Presentation of a decompressing manometer and autonomic bladder irrigator. *Journal of Urology* **11**: 373–394.

Tizes R (1981) Vasovagal syncope following rectal examination. *New York State Journal of Medicine* **81**(9): 1309–1310.

Whitteridge D (1960) Cardiovascular reflexes initiated from afferent sites other than the cardiovascular system itself. *Physiological Review* **30(supplement 4)**: 198.

12

Drop Attacks

INTRODUCTION

Drop attacks are an ambiguous condition, being both a symptom and a disease. They occur in association with such diverse diseases as parasagittal meningioma or narcolepsy and are predominantly a disease of middle-aged women. The **narcoleptic** drop attack (cataplexy) is almost always in response to sudden fear, anger, or uncontrollable laughing, associated with the rest of the narcoleptic disorder (although it may exist alone) and is therefore easily diagnosed.

Drop attacks are common in Britain but many North American neurolgists and internists will practice a lifetime and never meet an example. C. M. Fisher (personal communication) believes he has never seen it and the present author has a single patient with this diagnosis.

It was brought to prominence by Kremer (1958a, b) who wrote

> "a middle-aged person for no obvious reason falls where she stands. Most though not all patients are sure they do not lose consciousness. There is no warning, they do not try and save themselves because the whole episode is so sudden. They rise almost as soon as they reach the ground and are not confused. They are certain they do not trip, they felt well before the incident, and they feel well afterwards. Physical examination and investigations rarely reveal anything of note".

The term 'drop attack' was suggested by Kremer who has given an excellent clinical description of the syndrome in cases of injury of the cervical spine and in medullary compression. Sheehan *et al.* (1960) assumed the pathogenesis was sudden ischaemia of the pyramids in the region of the decussation. These are ventral in the medulla and lower brain-stem and supplied by the terminal branches of the vertebral artery including the anterior spinal arteries and first part of the basilar. The term 'drop attack' emphasized the sudden loss of posture due to paralysis of the legs, the reversibility of the attack and the maintenance of consciousness.

The description by Sheldon (1962) consisted of attacks in the elderly who suddenly and without warning would fall to the ground, without loss of consciousness and had no evidence of other disease. He thought the episodes were related to brain-stem and cerebellar cellular drop-out due to age, compounded by vertebral artery compression and postural hypotension.

Greenwood and Hopkins (1982) thought that the unifying factor between drop attacks, whatever the cause, might be failure of the ability of the quadriceps to generate tension quickly enough. They investigated the possibility that a delay in long loop (transcortical) reflexes might be responsible for the occurrence of drop attacks. Although unable to confirm this, they provided cogent arguments that in some subjects quadriceps tension cannot be generated fast enough to maintain the upright posture.

Further thoughtful papers on the subject have been contributed by Hallpike (1967) and Stevens and Matthews (1973).

Whatever the mechanism, Meissner *et al.* (1986) have followed 108 patients with this diagnosis for 6½ years. They defined a drop attack as a falling spell without warning or post-ictal complications with immediate righting and no loss of awareness. Information was obtained by subsequent examination, review of patient questionnaires and telephone interviews. Seventy-six women and 32 men met the definition. The mean age was 70 years and the average time from onset to diagnosis was three years.

Categories

Seven categories were defined:

1. *Unknown.* In 64% of the patients, there was no cause for drop attacks. Identifiable conditions in these patients, however, included peripheral vascular disease, diabetes, alcoholism, motor neurone disease, and Parkinsonism.

2. *Cardiovascular.* These patients (12%) had a history of cardiac disease and diagnosis was made on the basis of history and abnormalities in at least two of the following: cardiac examination, ECG, Holter monitoring and electrocardiography.

3. *Cerebrovascular disease.* In 7% there was a clear history of anterior or posterior cerebral circulation insufficiency, or both, separate from the drop attacks. Diagnosis was based on the history plus neurovascular examination, ocular blood pressure reading, head computed tomography scan or cerebral angiography.

4. *Combined cardiac–cerebrovascular disease.* (7%) Significant cardiac and cerebrovascular disease demonstrated by history, examination and diagnostic tests was noted.

5. *Seizure.* (5%) A history of active convulsive disorder associated with potentially epileptogenic activity on the EEG was present.

6. *Vestibular disease.* A history of labyrinthine dysfunction such as Ménière's disease or vertigo in the absence of vertebrobasilar ischaemic symptoms, occurred in 3%.

7. *Psychogenic.* The drop attack was witnessed by the examining neurologist and thought to be deliberate in 1%.

Prognosis and Survival

There was no difference in survival in the drop attack group and an age and sex-matched control population. Fifty-five patients (80%) of the group with no underlying mechanism, were symptom-free and half of them were untreated.

Three factors predicted poor survival: (a) a history of cardiac arrhythmia; (b) patients with an abnormal neurological examination; (c) a history of congestive heart failure. At follow-up, 92 of 108 patients were alive; 84% of untreated patients and 80% of the medically- or surgically-treated patients were free of symptoms. The falls had rarely caused injury.

Miessner *et al.* found no evidence that anaemia, spondylosis, degenerative cervical disc disease or hydrocephalus were important in the mechanism of the attacks.

Bilateral carotid occlusive disease or unilateral stenosis of a carotid supplying both anterior cerebral arteries may cause intermittent bilateral leg weakness and drop attacks. Cardiac disease or postural hypotension causing generalized hypoperfusion may aggravate haemodynamically-significant occlusive disease. One patient demonstrated a subclavian steal phenomenon and another had basilar artery occlusion.

A convulsive disorder involving the parasagittal cortex may be important. One patient demonstrated central midline movement activated paroxysmal fast activity associated with a sudden fall.

The drop attack is a relatively benign entity and prognosis is dictated by the other medical conditions the patient may have. If the cardiac and neurological examinations are negative the prognosis is favourable.

ASSOCIATED DISEASES

Epilepsy

In the International Classification of Seizures, epileptic drop attacks are classified as generalized and further described according to duration as 'epileptic drop attack' or 'atonic absence' or 'atonic seizure' (Gastaut, 1970, 1981).

Pazzaglia *et al.* (1985) describe the epileptic drop attack as a sudden, rapid, 'pure' fall without warning. The patient cannot protect himself and severe injury is common. There may be impairment of consciousness, the duration is one to two minutes, followed by brief confusion, and possible automatisms.

In a survey of 1200 epileptic patients seen over an eight-year-period, 16 were found to have drop attacks. The drop attack was never the first epileptic manifestation and appeared 1–30 years after the first seizure. The types of pre-existing seizures in these 16 patients were adversive, focal motor, partial complex or atypical absence.

The advent of the drop attack heralded a worsening of the patient's condition. This type of seizure is refractory to treatment, dangerous, and associated with a decay in the patient's personality and intellect. Clearly, these rare epileptic seizures are a manifestation of some progressive cerebral disease.

Tumours

Ethmoid, frontal and parasagittal tumours can cause attacks of lower extremity weakness while consciousness is preserved and these constitute a form of drop attack (Ethelberg, 1949, 1950).

Similar episodes occur in colloid cysts of the third ventricle (Kelly, 1951).

The tumour of the foramen magnum as described by Kremer (1958) may also be associated with attacks of sudden collapse of the legs.

Cataplexy

With or without narcolepsy and other components of the narcoleptic syndrome, cataplexy has been recognized as an episode which might drop the patient to his knees or onto the ground (Adie, 1926).

Labyrinthine and vestibulo-ocular dysfunction may cause drop attacks and must enter the differential diagnosis (Bental, 1979).

SPINAL CORD DISEASE

Ischaemia

Cord ischaemia from vertebrobasilar artery compression in cervical spondylosis or direct cord injury or anterior spinal artery lesions can all produce drop attacks (Sheehan *et al.*, 1960; Maurice-Williams, 1974).

In the extensive report on vertebral artery compression and cervical spondylosis by Sheehan *et al.* in 1960, the common symptoms were dizziness, vertigo, blurred vision, ataxia and drop attacks, usually on rotation or extension of the neck. They added a large number of patients in whom the signs and symptoms were precipitated by rotation or extension of the head and the pathogenesis was demonstrated during life.

Hind-brain Ischaemia; Parkinsonism

Lund (1965) found seven patients with drop attacks amongst 130 patients with syncope observed over a number of years. He defined the drop attack as coming on spontaneously and rapidly while the patient was standing or walking. They were not related to the start of walking, or moving or stopping, and generally were not associated with unconsciousness. Two of his seven patients had vertebrobasilar posterior cerebral artery system ischaemic symptoms; two others had Parkinsonism, and the fifth and sixth patients had both. In the seventh case no aetiology could be demonstrated. He agreed with Williams (1961) that drop attacks are most commonly a symptom of transient cerebral ischaemia in atherosclerosis of the vertebrobasilar artery system.

Syringomyelia and Hind-brain Herniation

Barnett *et al.* (1973) described two patients with communicating syringomyelia with drop attacks. In the first, the attacks were precipitated by head turning while in the second they were associated with headache. Neither patient lost consciousness and both were able to get back to their feet quickly and without complication.

Other patients with syringomyelia and the Arnold–Chiari malformation without syringomyelia have presented with drop attacks following coughing, head rotation or extension. Drop attacks plus occipital, neck and arm pain, or occipital headaches, would suggest atlanto-occipital disease as well. The attacks may occur in response to coughing, postural change or simply head extension or rotation.

Other Related Diseases

Finally, there are two common, treatable diseases which may present as drop attacks. Inter-

Table 12.1 Synopsis of drop attacks

- Drop attacks are most common in middle-aged women
- Up to 65% of patients with this symptom have no disease to account for it
- When a disease is present that explains the symptom it is most likely to be cardiovascular or cerebrovascular
- Less common diseases associated with drop attacks are parasagittal and foramen magnum intracranial tumours, syringomyelia and Arnold–Chiari malformation and seizure disorders

mittent complete heart block may send a standing patient crashing to the ground and there may be no clear historical report of clouding of consciousness or premonitoring light-headedness. The loss of the upright posture as a manifestation of global cerebral hypoxia in this situation without the more familiar symptoms is more likely to occur with complete heart block if one or more of the four major craniocervical vessels is occluded.

Unstable subluxations of the atlanto-axial joint in an advanced rheumatoid arthritic may be associated with abrupt and transient collapse with or without transient paresis of all four limbs.

The principal features of drop attacks are summarized in Table 12.1

REFERENCES

Adie WJ (1926) Idiopathic narcolepsy. A disease *sui generis* with remarks on the mechanism of sleep. *Brain* **49**: 257–306.

Barnett HJM, Foster JB and Hudgson P (1973) *Syringomyelia*, p. 21. London: W. B. Saunders.

Bental E and Hammond-Tooke GD (1979) Vertigo and drop attacks caused by acute transient monocular disequilibrium (Halpern's syndrome). *Journal of Neurology* **222**: 59–66.

Ethelberg S (1949) On cataplexy in a case of frontal lobe tumour. *Acta Psychologica Neurologica* **24**: 421–427.

Ethelberg S (1950) Symptomatic cataplexy or chalastic fits in cortical lesions of the frontal lobe. *Brain* **72**: 499–512.

Gastaut H (1970) Clinical and electroencephalographic classification of epileptic seizures. *Epilepsia* **11**: 102–113.

Gastaut H (1981) Proposal for revised clinical and electroencephalographic classification of epileptic seizures. *Epilepsia* **22**: 481–501.

Greenwood R and Hopkins A (1982) An attempt to explain the mechanism of drop attacks. *Journal of Neurological Science* **57**: 203–208.

Hallpike CS (1967) Discussion. In *Kinaesthetic and Vestibular Mechanisms (Ciba Foundation Symposium)* (eds AVS Reuck and JP Krieger) p. 190. London: Churchill.

Kelly R (1951) Colloid cysts of the third ventricle: analysis of 29 cases. *Brain* **74**: 23–65.

Kremer M (1958a) Sitting, standing, and walking. Part I. *British Medical Journal* **1**: 439–442.

Kremer M (1958b) Sitting, standing, and walking. Part II. *British Medical Journal* **2**: 121.

Lund M (1965) Drop attacks in association with Parkinsonism and basilar artery sclerosis. *Acta Neurologica Scandinavica* **39** (**supplement 14**): 226–229.

Maurice-Williams RS (1974) Drop attacks and cervical cord compression. *British Journal of Clinical Practice* **28**: 215–216.

Meissner I, Wibers DO, Swanson JW and O'Fallon WM (1986) The natural history of drop attacks. *Neurology* **36**: 1029–1034.

Pazzaglia P, D'Alessandro R, Ambrosetto G and Lugaresi E (1985) Drop attacks: an ominous change in the evolution of partial epilepsy. *Neurology* **35**: 1725–1730.

Sheehan S, Bauer RB and Meyer JS (1960) Vertebral artery compression in cervical spondylosis: arteriographic demonstration during life of vertebral artery insufficiency due to rotation and extension of the neck. *Neurology (Minneapolis)* **10**: 968–986.

Sheldon JH (1962) Drop attacks in the elderly. A request for information. *Journal of the College of General Practitioners* **5**: 107–109.

Stevens DL and Matthews WB (1973) Cryptogenic drop attacks. An affliction of women. *British Medical Journal* **1**: 439–442.

Williams D (1961) The syndromes of basilar insufficiency. In *Scientific Aspects of Neurology* (ed. H Garland). London: Livingstone.

13

Exercise and Syncope

NORMAL PHYSIOLOGY OF EXERCISE

Before exercise begins or at the start, there is increased sympathetic adrenergic activity to the heart and several vascular beds. This increases cardiac output, and produces vasoconstriction in non-exercising parts of the body and vasodilatation in the exercising muscles.

These are not exclusive exercise-related preparatory phenomenon. Emotional stress produces the same increased cardiac output, muscle blood flow and elevation of blood pressure.

Cortical, hypothalamic, as well as brainstem mechanisms for vasoconstriction, cardiac acceleration and vasodilatation are at work in the preparation for and in response to exercise. Baroreceptor responses which should inhibit some of these changes are overridden and the changes are permitted to continue.

A sedentary adult can increase his oxygen consumption to 10 times the resting level while exercising and a trained athlete can increase his oxygen consumption to 20 times the resting level (Little, 1985).

Muscle Blood Flow

During intense exercise, the huge increase in oxygen consumption by skeletal muscle is provided by an increase in muscle blood flow. This occurs from activation of cholinergic sympathetic vasodilator fibres. At the same time, stimulation of medullary sympathetic centres and inhibition of parasympathetic cardiac inhibitory centres leads to an increase in heart rate, cardiac output and peripheral vascular resistance (Little, 1985).

Increased muscle blood flow and the pumping action of exercising muscles increases venous return to the heart. The greater filling increases ventricular end-diastolic volume and cardiac stroke volume. The enhanced sympathetic discharge to the myocardium increases cardiac contractility.

There are further increases in heart rate, cardiac output and blood pressure from reflexes arising in active muscles and joints. Vasoactive metabolites from contracting muscles as well as autoregulation overcome sympathetic vasoconstrictor effects and *resistance vessels dilate.* This counteracts the central vasoconstrictor influences, a fall in total peripheral resistance occurs and blood is diverted to the active muscles. Flow may reach 20 times normal (Donald *et al.*, 1955).

In the working muscles, pre-capillary arterioles and under-perfused capillaries fill, increasing the surface area for interchange between blood and extracellular fluid. Capillary pressure in the active muscles remains high, assisting filtration. Muscular interstitial fluid and lymph flow increase and the circulating plasma volume may be reduced by as much as 10–12%. The shrinkage can be increased further by sweating.

Several hundred millilitres of blood may flow into muscle capillary beds at the start of active whole body exercise. This volume is large enough to compromise venous return and therefore constriction of the venous reservoir occurs. This is probably mediated through venous pressor receptors in the vena cava, right heart and pulmonary artery (Little, 1985).

Heart Function

The heart responds to exercise with an increase in rate and a larger stroke volume. The resulting output is in some ways related to the intensity of the muscular work and may be three or four times the resting level. The pulse rate can change very quickly and go as high as 150–175/min.

Initially the tachycardia is due to a reduction of vagal influences on the sino-atrial node and it persists in spite of an increase in blood pressure, suggesting an inhibition of the baroreceptor reflexes. Cardiac filling time is reduced as the rate increases. The contribution of venous return to increasing stroke volume diminishes with a tachycardia. Increased stroke volume is the larger contributor to increased cardiac output during light work, whereas the increase in rate is the major factor contributing to greater output with heavy work.

Blood Pressure

The blood-pressure response to exercise is related to the physical conditioning of the subject as well as the type of work performed. Isometric sustained hand grip at 50% of maximum strength causes a greater rise in blood pressure than the rhythmic, regular, exercise of running. Apparently the greater muscle mass involved in running and the greater general vasodilation in the vascular beds of these muscles compensates for the substantial rise in blood pressure seen when only a small amount of muscle mass is being used as in maximum hand grip. In human subjects, treadmill exercise produces a slight rise in systolic pressure and a fall in diastolic pressure. Whole-body exercise produces a generalized whole-body, muscle vascular-bed dilatation. Single muscle groups in static exercise produce relatively little vasodilatation and considerable vasoconstriction in the non-exercising parts of the body.

When exercise stops, pressure drops to resting levels or below and then returns towards its previous high level and then gradually declines. The transient fall in pressure following exercise probably has several causes. It is partially due to relaxation of abdominal muscles, reduced support of the venous reservoirs of the abdomen and thorax, with blood accumulating in the great veins and a drop in cardiac output.

In addition, at the end of exercise the pumping action of the muscles on their greatly increased vascular beds stops and there is some evidence to suggest that trained athletes are somewhat insensitive to the normal sympathetic responses initiated by a hypotensive period.

Coronary Blood Flow

When cardiac output increases three to four times the resting level, there is an appropriate increase in myocardial oxygen demand and therefore increased coronary blood flow. Of the increase in myocardial oxygen consumption during exercise the majority comes from increased coronary blood flow and a lesser amount from widening of the arterio-venous oxygen difference of the coronary circulation.

Pulmonary Circulation

There is an increase of the pulmonary vascular bed by the opening of new channels or expansion of already-perfused vascular channels, or both, during exercise. Pulmonary artery pressure remains below the upper limits of normal until the flow increases many times above the basal level. It then increases. The resistance in the pulmonary vascular bed initially decreases with exercise and pulmonary blood volume increases.

Respiratory Reflexes

Stretching the lung parenchyma in normal breathing as well as in exercise diminishes sympathetic vasoconstrictor tone to the skin, splanchnic and muscular vascular beds. This assists the re-distribution of blood flow to muscle. The hyperventilation practised by athletes before an event and accompanying strenuous exercise contributes to this increased muscle blood flow.

Body Temperature, Thermal Responses and Skin Blood Flow

Muscle work produces heat and an increase in temperature. This is excitatory to hypothalamic centres, with the result that vasoconstrictive sympathetic impulses to skin arterioles are inhibited. Cutaneous blood flow increases and heat is lost by convection and radiation from the skin. Initially this increases until the maximum work load is almost approached. The increase favours body cooling but further work causes a progressive decrease in skin flow as cutaneous sympathetic tone continues to rise. If the body temperature continues upward, sweating begins. This further inhibits the central venoconstriction of skin vessels and skin blood flow returns to normal or greater than normal. As a result, there is some diversion of blood from the muscles.

Figure 13.1 shows the major haemodynamic responses in exercising man, and the responses in a dog to both exercise and stimulation of the cardiac sympathetic fibres and the hypothalamic area. Figure 13.2 reveals the changes in regional distribution of cardiac output as the workload is increased.

EXCESS PARASYMPATHETIC TONE

Syncopal Athletes

Rasmussen *et al.* (1978) reported four patients aged 17, 23, 24 and 37 years of age with complaints of post-exercise syncope, repeated Adams–Stokes attacks, fatigue or dizziness at rest and periodic light-headedness and near syncope at rest. They were all exercising intensively between 10 and 30 h per week and had been doing so for up to 4 years. They were well-trained and the syncope was probably due to excess vagal tone. They had no evidence of cerebral or heart disease. They all had relative bradycardia, a constant finding in well-trained persons. The mechanisms are incompletely understood. Levy (1971) has suggested that it is an example of true reciprocal excitation. He believes that sympathetic impulses from work-

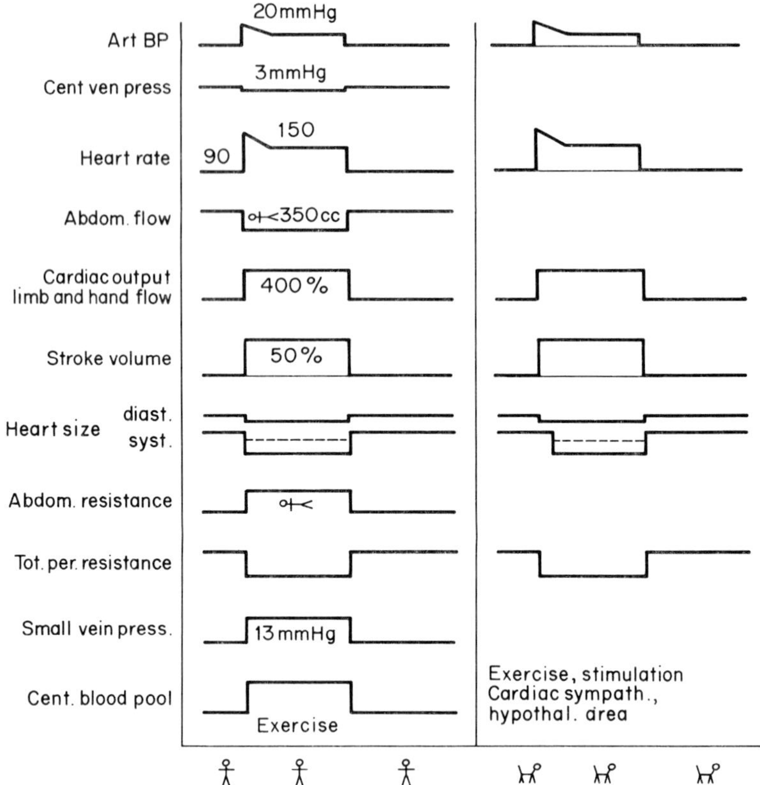

Figure 13.1 Haemodynamic changes in exercising man (left) and (right) the changes in an unanaesthetized dog from exercise and from stimulation of the cardiac sympathetic fibres and the hypothalamus. Unusual responses are shown (– – – – – – – –). (Reproduced with permission from Professor John B. West and *Best and Taylor's Physiological Basis of Medical Practice,* 10th Edition, 1978 (ed. J. R. Brobeck). Baltimore: The Williams and Wilkins Co.)

ing skeletal muscle provokes the release of acetylcholine from post-ganglionic vagal fibres by virtue of the action of norepinephrine at some presynaptic α-receptors.

The strong vagal tone caused by training improves the pumping capacity of the heart but during rest the vagal over-balance may be so marked that sino-atrial or atrioventricular block appears (Meytes *et al.,* 1975; Rasmussen *et al.,* 1978). A sick sinus node syndrome may be mimicked (Ferrer, 1973; Dighton, 1974; Rasmussen *et al.,* 1978).

The differentiation between physiological vagal depression of the sino-atrial node and a true sick sinus syndrome with structural changes may be based on sino-atrial node recovery time after rapid atrial pacing and the response to intravenous atropine. In two of Rasmussen's patients, abnormally long nodal recovery times were found after prolonged pacing. At rates higher than 120/min, a rate-dependent entrance block impeded over-drive suppression of the node. However, sino-atrial node function was normal after atropine in both patients.

Impairment of the atrioventricular node was present in all four patients but this also became normal after atropine.

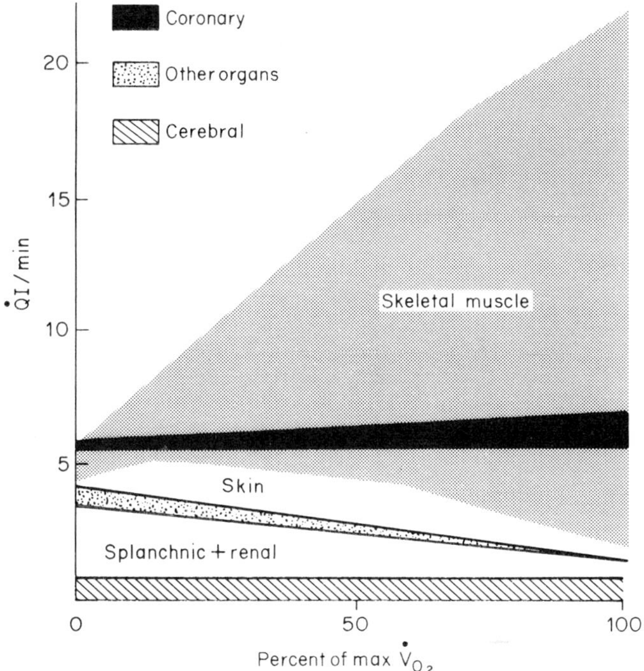

Figure 13.2 Regional changes in cardiac output as workload is increased.
Q = blood flow in litre per minute, V_{O_2} = oxygen consumption as a measure of the workload.
(Reproduced with permission from Professor John B. West and *Best and Taylor's Physiological Basis of Medical Practice,* 10th Edition, 1978 (ed. J. R. Brobeck). Baltimore: The Williams and Wilkins Co.)

From this study it is proposed that the bradycardia of athletes is an expression of vagal preponderance which suppresses all automatic and conductive tissues of the heart. In some cases the suppression is strong enough to provoke long sinus pauses at rest accompanied by cerebral symptoms. This risk is confined to periods of intensive training and ameliorated when training is stopped or the intensity is reduced.

A similar example has been described by Fleg and Asante (1983). Their patient, a 52-year-old man without evidence of organic heart disease by clinical and extensive non-invasive testing, had an 11-sec episode of asystole and unconsciousness 10 min *after* completing a maximum treadmill test. Four years earlier a similar episode had followed treadmill exercise.

Asystole with, or after, exercise testing is rare and not mentioned in two surveys with a total of about 170 000 exercise tests (Rochmis and Blackburn, 1971; Stuart and Ellestad, 1980).

This case demonstrates two important points. A post-exercise vagal reaction can be reproduced in a predisposed person, in this particular case after an interval of four years of good health. The asystolic episode was not in the early recovery period from exercise, but 10 min after the cessation of exercise.

Another aspect of autonomic dysfunction is less well-defined but nonetheless important, as reported in the small group of patients reported by Guilleminault *et al.* (1984). The four subjects, apparently healthy young adults, had vague histories of intermittent palpitations, chest pain radiating to the shoulder and light-headedness. The chest discomfort was generally unrelated to activity. One of them had two syncopal attacks after wakening to urinate. All four had normal electrocardiograms, echocardiograms, treadmill exercise tests and right-heart catheterization. Three of the four had left-heart catheterization and angiography, and all had normal haemodynamics. Electrophysiological studies in two demonstrated normal sinus-node and atrioventricular-node conduction. On 24-h ECG recordings, they all showed repeated episodes of asystole, with no evidence of escape rhythm during the daytime. None was syncopal and the longest sinus arrest varied from 7 to 9 sec. However, 95–98% of total cardiac arrhythmias occurred during sleep. In the daytime, the most common activities during which asystole occurred were exercise, urination and defaecation, exercise and sexual intercourse, and exercise and/or sexual intercourse in the fourth patient.

Polygraph recordings during sleep revealed no significant apnoeic episodes or decrease in oxygen saturation, but during REM sleep (in each case) 4–7 episodes of sinus arrest occurred lasting 2–6 sec.

The fact that REM sleep or a daytime activity known to be associated with changes in autonomic function was in every case associated with the asystolic periods suggests that the underlying pathophysiology involved autonomic dysfunction.

Apparently, adjustments in the autonomic nervous system occur during normal sleep involving both the sympathetic and parasympathetic systems. During sleep, the parasympathetic system is largely responsible for modulation of the heart rate (Mancia and Zanchetti, 1980).

Guilleminault *et al.* (1984) suggested that parasympathetic tone in his four patients was abnormally regulated and he chooses to support this by the predominance of asystole during REM sleep, urination, bowel movements or sexual intercourse.

Three of the four patients received ventricular inhibited pacemakers set at a lower rate limit of 40 beats/min. Two patients were asymptomatic for four and seven years with this therapy. It is recommended from this study that patients with day-time cardiac arrhythmias, thought to be secondary to abnormal vagal tone, should undergo 24-h Holter monitoring with the most thorough evaluation during sleep. In this way, one is more likely to document the occurrence of REM sleep-related cadiac dysrhythmias.

DIMINISHED SYMPATHETIC TONE

There is evidence of decreased sympathetic tone in endurance-trained subjects (Appenzeller *et al.*, 1985). The cold pressor test was used to evaluate the integrity and function of the sympathetic nervous system. They tested 43 subjects before and after a 49-km mountain race to an altitude of 3300 m. The subjects ranged from 21 to 56 years of age. They had an average increase of 7.6 mmHg systolic and 6.7 mmHg diastolic blood pressures in response to hand immersion in cold water before the race. After the race, the same test provoked a fall of 11.8 mmHg systolic and 3.3 mmHg in diastolic pressures. These differences are significant.

Endurance-trained subjects are known to have enhanced parasympathetic tone and this observation of Appenzeller *et al.* indicates an attenuation of sympathetic tone as well. The implications are that either the central mechanisms or efferent fibre functions related to cold-induced sympathetic reflex vasoconstriction are impaired after prolonged exercise in these subjects.

POST-EXERTIONAL ORTHOSTATIC FAINTING

Brogdon and Hellebrandt (1940), Eichna and Bean (1944), and others have documented orthostatic hypotension following hard muscular work. The phenomenon is transient and usually a non-fatal collapse.

The physiological changes in healthy young men, worked to their limits, and then examined while in the post-exertional orthostatic hypotensive state were studied by Eichna *et al.* (1947). After the exercise all subjects were placed upright for two 5-min periods, separated by one 5-min supine period.

Results

The subjects were categorized as syncopal, abnormal and normal. The syncopal group developed syncope and were unable to remain erect for 5 min during either or both of the two erect periods after exercise. While erect they had low blood pressure and rapid pulse. Their symptoms when upright were apprehension nausea, abdominal cramps and dizziness. These were accompanied by dimness of vision, vomiting, disorientation and unconsciousness. Just prior to unconsciousness the pulse slowed remarkably in a number of subjects. On being placed in the supine position, all symptoms improved or disappeared and the subject recovered. Immediately after becoming supine a marked bradycardia and elevation of blood pressure were encountered.

The abnormal group included those who were able to remain erect for 5 min during both erect periods without syncope, but during one of these they sustained a blood pressure below 100 mmHg. Many developed symptoms and signs similar to the syncopal group but did not become syncopal.

The normal group all remained erect, without symptoms, and with systolic blood pressures above 100 mmHg.

In 19 of 33 subjects, there was development of post-exertional orthostatic hypotension after exhausting physical work; 9 became syncopal and 10 did not. The syncope was likely to occur when systolic pressure fell to 80 mmHg. Pulse pressure bore less relationship. Syncope was more likely in the second erect period (15 min after the cessation of exercise) than in the first erect period (5 min after the work). The blood pressure was identical in all three groups—normal, abnormal and syncopal—when supine. Tachycarda accompanied the hypotension but the heart slowed just as collapse occurred. In one instance cardiac slowing progressed to asystole of 19 sec.

The duration of the post-exertional orthostatic hypotension varied. In one subject it was present 1 h after stopping work and it was $1\frac{1}{4}$ h after the exertion before he could remain erect for 5 min. In general, there was recovery from syncope within 1 h and from hypotension in the abnormal group in 2 h.

There are no predictive physical characteristics related to the subjects and their tendency to cardiovascular collapse.

Repeat testing with repetition of the work on subsequent days showed improvement and even disappearance of the post-exertional orthostatic hypotension and syncope so that adaptation does occur. Similarly, repeated testing of the abnormal group failed to produce hypotension in 50% of the group on the second test. There was no difference in cardiovascular responses to the cold pressor test or mental arithmetic between the groups.

Mechanism of the Hypotension

With the trunk erect and the legs horizontal (sitting) the blood pressure rose. The hypotension persisted, but was not severe enough to cause syncope which recurred when the legs were lowered again to the dependent position.

During the orthostatic hypotension even passive movement of the fully dependent legs caused the blood pressure to rise.

If, before tilting the subject erect, the circulation of both legs was occluded with inflated blood pressure cuffs to 240 mmHg, orthostatic hypotension did not occur, but developed rapidly in preceding and subsequent erect periods without the thigh cuffs.

Orthostatic hypotension developed in approximately one-half of normal young men following vigorous exercise of the legs. It occurred after prolonged moderate work as well as acute exhausting work. In half of those who developed orthostatic hypotension, it was severe enough to produce syncope. The pooling of blood in the legs, presumably due to failure of muscular venous pumping plus a dilatation of vascular beds, is responsible. During the orthostatic hypotension, if blood was moved out of the legs or blood was excluded from them, the hypotension was relieved.

Exertional Hypotension

Exertional hypotension may result in patients with varied cardiac disorders as described by Bruce (1959), including severe coronary artery stenosis (Levites *et al.*, 1978). Normal subjects free of all heart disease may develop exertional hypotension following maximal, exhaustive, exercise.

Tsutsumi and Hara (1979) described the following patient.

> *Case study.* The patient had mild ischaemic heart disease and subsequently developed syncopal episodes after running, and hypotension plus bradycardia after exercise. He was a 48-year-old, well-trained soldier. Seven years earlier he had had episodes of syncope while standing after running 2 km. He was symptom-free while running, but fainted when he suddenly stopped running. Two years earlier he had had an abnormal ECG suggesting ischaemic heart disease but had no chest pain, palpitations or shortness of breath even after running. He was on no medication, had a blood pressure of 100/58 mmHg in each arm, no orthostatic hypotension, a grade-II systolic murmur at the apex, normal peripheral vessels and a normal neurological examination.
>
> Cardiac catheterization, left ventriculogram, and left ventricle end-diastolic pressures were normal, while coronary angiography revealed 50% stenosis of the left circumflex artery close to its origin, and 25% stenosis of the right coronary artery.
>
> Direct brachial artery pressure measurements showed a fall in blood pressure from 152/64 mmHg during exercise to 100/40 mmHg immediately after exercise. This level persisted for 10–15 cardiac cycles, and after a short-lived increase it fell again to 80/12 mmHg with bradycardia for about a minute. During this time he was light-headed without syncope.
>
> The fall of blood pressure after exercise could be prevented by giving a β-adrenergic blocking agent (pindolol) 20 mg orally.

His valsalva manoeuvre, cold-pressor test and mental arithmetic test, were normal. Plasma norepinephrine, epinephrine and dopamine were respectively 260, 25 and 115 ng/litre in the supine position and 706, 98 and 278 ng/litre in the upright position after 10 min (normal). Blood gases, plasma lactate and pyruvate values before and after exercise were normal.

There are two points of view concerning the mechanism of this clinical situation. Thomson and Keleman (1975) believed that a fall in systolic pressure during exercise was a sign of severely compromised left-ventricular blood supply. In contrast, Levites *et al.* (1978) found hypotension during exercise in only 2.7% of the paients they tested and the extent and distribution of their coronary disease was no different from those patients with a normal blood-pressure response during exercise. In their patients, the hypotension occurred during, and not after, the exercise.

In the patient described by Tsutsumi and Hara the hypotension was after exercise. The coronary artery narrowing was unreleated to the syncope. His normal valsalva response indicated an intact baroreceptor reflex arc. The vasodepressor, bradycardia syncope associated with the end of exercising and prevented with a β-blocker, suggested that the syncope was caused by β-receptor-mediated neurogenic peripheral vasodilatation.

WEIGHTLIFTER'S BLACKOUT

Compton *et al.* (1973) have studied weightlifter's blackout. They examined weightlifters performing the 'clean-and-jerk' lift. In this event, the competitor lifts the bar-bell from the floor to a position across the front of his neck, the 'clean'. He first hyperventilates, squats, performs a valsalva, lifts the bar to hip height as he stands, semi-squats again and lifts the bar to neck height and then straightens his posture. In the 'jerk' phase he takes a stride with both knees and both hips slightly flexed, repeates the valsalva, lifting the bar from the neck to above the head, then brings the feet back together and the lift is complete. At this point he may faint.

There is vigorous and lengthy hyperventilation at the start which decreases cerebral perfusion. Muscle vascular beds are dilated. Then there is a prolonged squatting adding to peripheral vasodilatation, temporarily reducing peripheral resistance and venous return. Raised intrathoracic pressure is added and may be as high as 160–260 mmHg in professional weightlifters. This intrathoracic pressure is transmitted to central vessels and to the arterial pulse pressure. It also obstructs venous return, and cardiac volume, stroke volume and pulse pressure begin to fall. At the end of the valsalva the transmitted intrathoracic pressure is released and arterial pressure falls rapidly. Simultaneously, the great veins, the splanchnic vessels and probably the pulmonary vessels, previously compressed by the high intrathoracic pressure, expand. Filling of these causes a lag in the transit of blood to the left ventricle so that for a few beats output is severely reduced or even abolished.

The peripheral arterial resistance is also low. Then a repetition of the valsalva manoeuvre for the next stage of the lift re-imposes the abnormalities before recovery has occurred from the first round. The syncope results from cerebral ischaemia produced by a transient fall in arterial pressure when the raised intrathoracic pressure is released. Cine-angiography has demonstrated the delay in the ventricular filling at the release of the high intrathoracic pressure and blood pressure fell transiently to 25–50 mmHg.

REFERENCES

Appenzeller O, Appenzeller J, Skipper B and Snyder R (1985) Attenuation of cold pressor test: evidence for decreased sympathetic tone in endurance-trained subjects. *Annals of Neurology* **18**(1): 150–151.

Best and Taylor's Physiological Basis of Medicine (1978), 10 Edition (ed. JR Brobeck). Baltimore: The Williams and Wilkins Company.

Brogdon E and Hellebrandt FA (1940) Post-exercise orthostatic collapse. *American Journal of Physiology* **129**: 318.

Bruce RA, Leonard, AC, Shigeaki K, Morledge JH, Andrus WW and Fuller TJ (1959) Exertional hypotension in cardiac patients. *Circulation* **19**: 543–551.

Compton D, Hill PM and Sinclair JD (1973) Weightlifter's blackout. *Lancet* **2**(840): 1234–1237.

Dighton DH (1974) Sinus bradycarda. Autonomic influences and clincal assessment. *British Heart Journal* **36**: 791

Donald KW, Bishop JM, Cumming G and Wade OL (1955) The effect of exercise on the cardiac output and circulatory dynamics of normal subjects. *Clinical Science* **14**: 37–73.

Eichna LW and Bean WB (1944) Orthostatic hypotension in normal young men following physical exertion, environmental thermal loads, or both. *Journal of Clinical Investigation* **23**: 942 (abstract).

Eichna LW, Horvath SM and Bean WB (1947) Post exertional orthostatic hypotension. *American Journal of Medical Sciences* **213**: 641–654

Ferrer I (1973) The sick sinus syndrome. *Circulation* **47**: 635.

Fleg JL and Asante AV (1983) Asystole following treadmill exercise in a man with organic heart disease. *Archives of Internal Medicine* **143**(9): 1821–1822.

Guilleminault C, Pool P, Motta J and Gillis AM (1984) Sinus arrest during REM sleep in young adults. *New England Journal of Medicine* **311**(16): 1006–1010.

Levites R, Baker T and Anderson GJ (1978) The significance of hypotension developing during treadmill exercise testing. *American Heart Journal* **95**: 747–753.

Levy MN (1971) Sympathetic–parasympathetic interactions in the heart. *Circulation Research* **29**: 437.

Little RC (1985) *Physiology of the Heart and Circulation*, 3rd Edition. Chicago: Year Book Medical Publishers.

Mancia G and Zanchetti A (1980) Cardiovascular regulation during sleep. In *Physiology in Sleep* (eds J Orem and C Barnes) pp. 2–54. New York: Academic Press.

Meytes I, Kaplinsky E, Yahini JH, Hanne-Paparo N and Neufeld HN (1975) Wenchebach AV block. A frequent feature following heavy physical training. *American Heart Journal* **90**: 426.

Rasmussen V, Haunso S and Skagen K (1978) Cerebral attacks due to excessive vagal tone in heavily trained persons. *Acta Medica Scandinavica* **204**: 401–405.

Rochmis P and Blackburn H (1971) Exercise tests, a survey of procedures, safety, and litigation experience in approximately 170 000 tests. *Journal of the American Medical Association* **217**: 1061–1066.

Stuart RJ and Ellestad MH (1980) National survey of exercise and stress testing facilities. *Chest* **77**: 94–97.

Thomson PD and Keleman MH (1975) Hypotension accompanying the onset of exertional angina. A sign of severe compromise of left ventricular blood supply. *Circulation* **52**: 28–32.

Tsutsumi E and Hara H (1979) Syncope after running. *British Medical Journal* **2**(6203): 1480.

14

Mastocytosis and Other Disorders

MASTOCYTOSIS

Mastocytosis is an abnormal proliferation of tissue mast cells in multiple organs. Symptoms have been attributed to the release of histamine. However, a combination of H_1- and H_2-receptor blocking agents is ineffective in preventing the recurrent life-threatening episodes of flushing and hypotension characteristic of this disease.

Roberts *et al.* (1982) have found that in addition to histamine there is also a marked overproduction of prostaglandin D_2 (PGD_2).

The diagnostic hallmark has been the presence of *urticaria pigmentosa* as 99% of patients with the disease are said to have this cutaneous lesion.

Clinical Mastocytosis

Symptoms. These are protean and a consequence of the paroxysmal release of mast-cell mediators. They occur in a wide variety of combinations and rarely does one patient have them all. Included in the very common ones by Roberts *et al.* (1982) are flushing, palpitations, dizziness, syncope, chest pain, headaches, intermittent diarrhoea, chronic fatigue and dyspnoea without wheezing.

Central Nervous System Dysfunction

The single most common symptom is episodic flushing; however, the sudden release of mast-cell mediators may depress the blood pressure so quickly that flushing never occurs or only as the hypotensive and syncopal crisis is over.

The female:male relationship is 4:1 and the mean age is 45 years. The disease is episodic and the attacks culminate in syncope while the less-severely affected have dizziness. Flushing is of universal occurrence and not often a volunteered symptom. Itchiness is extremely common, usually chronic, although it may occur only during attacks. Palpitation, tachycardia and headaches are frequent and also may occur only during attacks. Most patients have intermittent abdominal cramps and diarrhoea.

During an attack, shortness of breath, paraesthesiae, nausea and vomiting, chest pain and vertigo, are all common. A family history of similar symptoms is common and almost all patients demonstrate a wheal-and-flare on stroking the skin. Most patients find their symptoms exacerbated by exertion, anxiety and heat.

It has been established that a PGD_2 urinary metabolite is increased up to as much as 150-fold above normal. The PGD_2 production may be abated by daily aspirin and aspirin plus antihistamine are even more effective. The most effective drugs in the experience of Roberts *et al.* (1982) are chlorpheniramine, cimetidine and aspirin.

Urticaria pigmentosa is not necessary for diagnosis as the essence of the disease is the release of histamine and PGD_2 producing pulmonary vascular constriction and systemic vasodilatation leading to syncope.

In another report, Roberts (1984) stated that attacks could occur at the rate of one or two per month and be associated with episodic loss of consciousness for 30–60 min. Skin biopsy revealed mast-cell hyperplasia with 12–18 mast cells per high-power field, the normal being six. Mastocytosis can be a localized or a systemic disease and there is a small group of patients with the classical symptoms but increased cell proliferation cannot be found. The most common form of localized mastocytosis is limited to the skin. A solitary mastocytoma occurs almost exclusively in children and responds well to excision.

In systemic mastocytosis bony abnormalities, osteoporosis, or osteosclerosis, hepatosplenomegaly, gastrointestinal mucosal nodules, anaemia, leucocytosis or mast cell leukaemia may occur (Roberts, 1984).

Agents known to evoke mast-cell activation and to be avoided are narcotic analgesics, radiological contrast media, alcohol and muscle relaxants. Non-steroidal anti-inflammatory drugs, β-adrenergic receptor antagonists, α-adrenergic receptor agonists and cholinergic receptor agonists, are all mast-cell activators and should be avoided. A small percentage of patients with mastocytosis are sensitive to aspirin and this or any non-steroidal anti-inflammatory drug can evoke severe bronchospasm. Epinephrine, which can reverse the severe vasodilatory hypotension in mastocytosis, is an important drug in this disease and β-receptor antagonists are clearly contraindicated. Roberts has encountered patients with the disease in whom attacks with syncope occurred only during β-receptor antagonist therapy.

HOLMES–ADIE SYNDROME

Croll *et al.* (1935) reported orthostatic hypotension in a patient with Holmes–Adie syndrome. Johnson *et al.* (1971) reported two patients with orthostatic hypotension and this syndrome. One, aged 50 years, reported giddiness and light-headedness on walking briskly or on standing after sitting or stooping. He had a past history of epilepsy although his EEG was normal. The second patient, aged 20 years, had vertigo on rising from sitting to standing and complained that the dizziness was accompanied by widespread sweating. Both patients had reduced or absent tendon stretch reflexes and asymmetrical pupils which reacted slowly to light with a sluggish unilateral response to accommodation.

Investigations suggested they both had an afferent baroreceptor block.

PORPHYRIA

Schirger *et al.* (1962) reported a 47-year-old woman with orthostatic hypotension associated with an acute exacerbation of porphyria. The hypotension was treated by the use of head-up bed tilt. The severity of the postural hypotension diminished as the symptoms of the peripheral neuropathy lessened. Exacerbation of the porphyria followed renewed exposure to toxic agents and the orthostatic hypotension worsened concurrently.

PRIMARY ALDOSTERONISM

Okubo *et al.* (1977) reported a 27-year-old patient with primary aldosteronism presenting as syncopal attacks. The cause of the syncope was attributable to ventricular tachyarrhythmia which in turn was due to hypokalaemia. A similar case of hyperaldosteronism presenting with repetitive Adams–Stoke attacks was reported by Morton and Bekheit (1970).

CRANIOPHARYNGIOMA

Thomas *et al.* (1961) reported a 52-year-old man with orthostatic hypotension as the presenting sign of a craniopharyngioma. They believe that any patient with orthostatic hypotension should be investigated for an intracranial lesion. Parasellar and intrasellar tumours may manifest themselves by disturbance of orthostatic blood-pressure regulation. This patient had hypotension for two years prior to the diagnosis. Surgical removal of the tumour did not alter the orthostatic hypotension.

MYASTHENIA GRAVIS

Maclean and Horton (1937) reported a 46-year-old man with autonomic failure, postural hypotension and myasthenia gravis.

VILLOUS ADENOMA AND HYPONATRAEMIA

Jeanneret-Grosjean *et al.* (1978) described a case with major fluid and electrolyte depletion due to a large villous adenoma. The diagnosis was delayed because of a nearly normal serum potassium and the impression that hyponatraemia is not a feature of villous adenoma. In villous adenoma of the colon, loss of water, sodium, chloride and potassium all occur.

> *Case study*. The patient described by Jeanneret-Grosjean *et al.* was an 82-year-old female complaining of the passage of 'urine per rectum' for the previous six years and repeated attacks of unconsciousness. She was thought to have transient cerebral ischaemic attacks. After the appropriate biochemical assessment it was evident that the syncopal attacks were due to hyponatraemia, hypovolaemia and postural hypotension. She was secreting a rectal fluid volume of 1500 ml in 24 h with a high sodium and potassium content. With resection of the large benign villous adenoma the watery discharge ended, the fainting spells and postural hypotension disappeared, electrolytes remained normal and the patient recovered.

UNDERWATER FAINTING—A MECHANISM OF DROWNING

In an attempt to extend underwater swimming time, swimmers hyperventilate before going into the water. They may lose consciousness before the desire to breathe is overwhelming and they can then drown. Dumitru and Hamilton (1964) reported two examples. Both survived and both reported that just prior to unconsciousness they had no panic or urgency with respect to breathing.

Hyperventilating for a few minutes before swimming can increase alveolar oxygen tension to 140 mmHg and diminish carbon dioxide tension to 15 mmHg. The arterial blood oxygen increase is negligible while the reduced carbon dioxide content is significant. The latter produces cerebral vasoconstriction and can reduce cerebral blood flow by one-third. Even if there was a concurrent rise of arterial oxygen tension, the hypocapnoea reduces oxygen dissociation from haemoglobin and less oxygen is available.

As the tissue oxygen is utilized during swimming the contracting muscles continue to function and accumulate an oxygen debt. As the oxidative metabolism of glucose diminishes less carbon dioxide is formed with increased production of lactic acid.

In the brain, glucose must be completely oxidized for its efficient utilization. With reduced oxygen available the energy yield does not supply cellular demands. The diminished oxidative metabolism of glucose further reduces carbon dioxide production, compounding the abnormal cerebral metabolism.

A third factor is the rigid chest posture maintained by the underwater swimmer. This is a valsalva manoeuvre which produces a fall in systemic arterial pressure further compounding the cerebral hypoxia.

Diving bradycardia can be a factor in underwater syncope (Bove *et al.* 1973). They studied heart rate during prolonged breath-holding with the face immersed. Bradycardia immediately after facial immersion occurred in all subjects. In four, a second decline in heart rate occurred after about 140 sec of breath-holding and continued until breathing was resumed. The secondary decline was thought to be due to hypoxia developing during prolonged apnoea in individuals who can better tolerate hypoxia and hypercapnoea. These individuals may be more prone to sudden underwater blackout during breath-holding dives. Their initial diving bradycardia is later potentiated by the progressive hypoxia which further reduces cardiac output and blood flow to vital organs.

BRAIN DISEASES THAT CAUSE HEART DISEASE AND MAY CAUSE SYNCOPE

Smaje *et al.* (1987) reported a well-documented case of sino-atrial arrest due to temporal lobe epilepsy. Autonomic events may accompany many types of epileptic seizures. They can occur as a normal response to the stress of the attack but may also result from seizure activity spreading to autonomic centres. Alterations in heart rate or rhythm are among the possible causes of death during a seizure. Tachyarrhythmias are more common than bradyarrhythmias. There are possibly only three documented cases of sino-atrial arrest in association with temporal lobe epilepsy (Phizackerly *et al.*, 1954; Katz *et al.*, 1983).

The case reported by Smaje *et al.* is as follows.

> *Case study.* The patient was a 35-year-old male whose attacks consisted of *déjà vu* at which time his pulse was between 50 and 60 per minute. In the next 15 sec there was a

progressive bradycardia leading to asystole for a further 20 sec, loss of consciousness and some twitching of the limbs. Atropine returned his heart rate to normal and he had five similar attacks before a cardiac pacemaker was inserted. His ECG between attacks was normal, clinical examination was normal, and his EEG showed left temporal, irregular, slow activity. The pacemaker was removed and monitoring showed occasional second-degree heart block (Wenkebach phenomenon) at night only. He was discharged on phenytoin, the seizures continued, and eventually because of headache and right optic atrophy, a right epidermoid tumour adherent to the optic chiasm and undersurface of the hypothalmus and frontal lobes on the right was diagnosed and removed. There were no further seizures or syncope.

In the two other patients who have had simultaneous EEG and ECG monitoring, sino-atrial arrest during temporal lobe seizures was found. The asystole occurred shortly after the seizure onset and lasted for 8–10 sec, prior to the development of a generalized convulsion.

Jay and Lesstma (1981) have suggested that a significant cardiac arrhythmia caused by a primary epileptic disturbance may be more common than is generally supposed and urged combined ECG and EEG monitoring.

Reinstein *et al.* (1972) reported that 60% of patients with stroke had arrhythmias in the three days after the event while Lavy *et al.* (1974) found arrhythmias in half of the patients with ischaemic stroke and 78% of patients with haemorrhagic stroke. Joynt and Feibel (1982) observed high levels of catecholamines in these patients compared to those without arrhythmia.

Reich *et al.* (1981) examined the histories of patients after recovery from episodes of arrhythmia. They found that 20% experienced acute emotional upset in the 24 h prior to the arrhythmia and in nearly two-thirds of the cases the emotional distress preceded the onset of ventricular tachycardia or fibrillation by less than 1 h. Lown and DeSilva (1978) found that psychological stress could increase the number of ventricular ectopic beats in 11 of 19 patients. Alterations of autonomic activity by carotid massage, valsalva manoeuvre, breath holding, etc. accomplished this in only one of this group.

Finally, in the prolonged Q–T syndrome (see Chapter 8), in which children have paroxysmal ventricular arrhythmias which are potentially lethal, stress as well as physical exertion is commonly acknowledged to precipitate attacks. Clearly, many kinds of central nervous system activity and disease can change the level of cardiac function which in turn can lead to paroxysmal episodes of unconsciousness or syncope.

The trauma of pneumo-encephalography can provoke syncope. Polygraph recordings, EEG and ECG, intraspinal and intra-arterial pressures, were recorded during pneumo-encephalograms by Oftedal (1967). A large number of patients fainted and some of these attacks were vasovagal with bradycardia, diminished blood and CSF pressures. However, some patients fainted with no change in heart rate. blood pressure or intraspinal pressure. The EEG showed bilateral slowing and many patients had cardiac irregularities; a few of them had asystole for up to 20 sec.

The trauma to the brain of the CSF-oxygen exchange has some direct effect on the regulation of cardiac rate and conduction.

POST-OPERATIVE LEAKING THECA AND ORTHOSTATIC SYNCOPE

Marlin (1980) reported a 14-year-old girl with diastematomyelia. After surgery, which was otherwise successful, she developed a pseudomeningocele. She complained of intermittent, sub-occipital, headache and occasional syncopal episodes only when upright. The pseudomeningocele of approximately 500 ml of CSF was resolved when several large holes in the dura were closed.

Klein *et al.* (1963) also reported the following case.

> *Case study.* A patient had postural syncope due to a post-operative lumbar meningocele. This patient had a herniated lumbar intravertebral disc removed and four years later a second operation to remove spinal adhesions in the lumbar area. She then had wound dehiscence, discharge of a large amount of CSF, and shortly thereafter began to have episodes of severe headache, emesis, a throbbing sensation in the head, dimness of vision and loss of consciousness. These attacks occurred 2–4 times a day and lasted about 30 sec. They were always associated with a change in posture: sitting up in bed, standing erect, and could be avoided by rising slowly and walking with her head and shoulders bent forward. Straightening the spine almost always resulted in a loss of consciousness. Syncope was usually followed by a severe headache and backache.
>
> She had a 15-cm midline mass in the lumbar region at the site of the previous surgery and the valsalva manoeuvre produced a visible and palpable increase in size and tension of the mass. The meningocele was closed surgically. Her pulse and blood pressure were insignificantly changed when she was tilted from supine to 45° head up, in which position she became unconscious.

REFERENCES

Bove AA, Pierce AL, Barrera F, Amsbaugh GA and Lynch PR (1973) Diving bradycardia as a factor in underwater blackout. *Aerospace Medicine* **44**(3): 245–248.

Croll WF, Duthie RJ and MacWilliam JA (1935) Postural hypotension: report of a case. *Lancet* **1**: 194–198.

Dumitru AP and Hamilton LG (1964) Underwater blackout, a mechanism of drowning. *General Practitioner* **29**: 123–125.

Jay GW and Lesstma JE (1981) Sudden death in epilepsy: a comprehensive review of the literature and proposed mechanisms. *Acta Neurologica Scandinavica* **63(supplement 82)**: 1–66.

Jeanneret-Grosjean AJ, Tse GN and Thompson WG (1978) Villous adenoma with hyponatremia and syncope. *Diseases of Colon and Rectum* **21**(2): 118–119.

Johnson RH, McLellan DL and Love DR (1971) Orthostatic hypotension and the Holmes–Adie syndrome. *Journal of Neurology, Neurosurgery and Psychiatry* **34**: 562–570.

Joynt RJ and Feibel JH (1982) Stroke: another view. *Perspectives in Biological Medicine* **26**: 116–126.

Katz RI, Tiger M and Harner RN (1983) Epileptic cardiac arrhythmia: sino-atrial arrest in two patients. A potential cause of sudden death in epilepsy. *Epilepsia* **24**: 248.

Klein LJ, Woodhall B and Heyman A (1963) Acute reduction in intracranial pressure as a mechanism of postural syncope in a patient with post-operative lumbar meningocele. *Neurology (Minneapolis)* **13**: 146–151.

Lavy S, Yaar I, Melamed E *et al.* (1974) Effect of acute stroke on cardiac function as observed in an intensive stroke care unit. *Stroke* **5**: 775–780.

Lown B and DeSilva RA (1978) Roles of psychological stress and autonomic nervous system changes in provocation of ventricular premature complexes. *American Journal of Cardiology* **41**: 979–985.

MacLean AR and Horton BT (1937) Myasthenia gravis with postural hypotension. *Proceedings of Staff Meeting Mayo Clinic* **12**: 787–792.

Marlin AE (1980) Positional headache and syncope associated wtih pseudomeningocele. *Archives of Neurology* **37**(11): 736–737.

Morton P and Pekheit S (1970) Hyperaldosteronism presenting with repetitive Stokes–Adams attacks. *Irish Journal of Medical Sciences* **3**: 357–361.

Oftedal SI (1967) Polygraphic recordings during syncope. *Electroencephalography and Clinical Neurophysiology* **22**: 392.

Okubo S, Hiejima K, Satake S and Sakamoto Y (1977) Syncope as a manifestation of primary aldosteronism. *Archives of Internal Medicine* **137**(9): 1260.

Phizackerly PJR, Poole EW and Whitty CWM (1954) Sino-auricular heart block as an epileptic manifestation. *Epilepsia* **3**: 89–91.

Reich P, DeSilva RA and Lown B (1981) Acute psychological disturbances preceding life-threatening ventricular arrhythmias. *Journal of the American Medical Association* **246**: 233–235.

Reinstein L, Gravey JG, Kline JA *et al.* (1972) Cardiac monitoring of the acute stroke patient. *Archives of Physical Medicine Rehabilitation* **53**: 311–314.

Roberts LJ (1984) Recurrent syncope due to systemic mastocytosis. *Hypertension* **6**(2) (part 1): 285–294.

Roberts LJ, Fields JP and Oates JA (1982) Mastocytosis without urticaria pigmentosa. A frequently unrecognized cause of recurrent syncope. *Transactions of the Association of American Physicians* **95**: 36–41.

Schirger A, Martin WJ, Goldstein NP and Hunzinga KA (1962) Orthostatic hypotension in association with acute exacerbation of porphyria. *Proceedings of Staff Meeting Mayo Clinic* **37**: 7–11.

Smaje JC, Davidson C and Teasdale GM (1987) Sino-atrial arrest due to temporal lobe epilepsy. *Journal of Neurology, Neurosurgery and Psychiatry* **50**(1): 112–113.

Thomas JE, Schirger A, Love JG and Hoffman DL (1961) Orthostatic hypotension as the presenting sign in craniopharyngioma. *Neurology (Minneapolis)* **11**: 418–423.

Index